MS
Living Symptom Free

The True Story of an MS Patient

by Daryl H. Bryant

A Guide on How to Eat Properly and Live a Healthy Life While Controlling, Reducing, and Eliminating the Symptoms of Multiple Sclerosis

Includes over Twenty-Five MS-friendly Recipes

MS - Living Symptom Free

For additional copies of this publication, please visit www.MSLivingSymptomFree.com

Printed in the United States of America

First Printing: August 2011

Copyright © 2011 Daryl H Bryant

ISBN: 0615467016
ISBN-13: 9780615467016
LCCN: 2011925907

To my amazing wife Shannon

who has always been there

with love and support.

Table of Contents

Introduction

Are you or someone you love and care for living with Multiple Sclerosis (MS)? MS can be a devastating disease that can turn everything in your life upside down. For many people the struggle to discover a happier, healthier way to live with the disease can seem like an impossible task. It is important for you and others with MS to realize is that it *is* possible.

In this book, you will learn a great deal about my story of personal success in living, loving, and enjoying my life as an MS patient. I am not a doctor—simply a patient whose experience has run the gamut of emotion when it comes to MS. While today I'm a happy, healthy person who is able to manage the symptoms of this condition, I was not that person when I was first diagnosed. Instead, it took hitting absolute rock bottom, mired in pain and depression for quite some time, before I became the healthy and happy person I am today. I want to share my success story with you in the hopes that it will make your journey easier.

Understand that pain, worry, and a sense of struggle are completely natural for people living with MS. You are not alone in this disease. This book is here to help you realize this and to assist you in learning what you can do to start a new, healthier, and happier life. MS is a lifelong condition, but it doesn't have to control your life. With the right changes, you can help conquer the symptoms of this disease and put control of your life back into your own hands.

It is my hope that my story will offer you inspiration and remind you that there are others out there battling this disease and winning. No two cases of MS are exactly alike, but I hope you can use my story, my symptoms, and my successes to help you make the changes you need to achieve better health. It can be done; you can live a healthier and happier life with MS.

About the Author

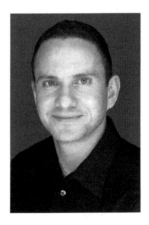

I was born on May 23, 1977 to loving and fantastic parents. I have an older sister and we lived in Byram, a small rural town in New Jersey.

I was very active during my childhood and teenage years; I loved sports and participated in football, basketball, karate, wrestling, and tap dancing to name a few. I've also enjoyed golf, Jiu-Jitsu, hunting, and more. I loved being active and playing sports, whether the game was played alone or with a team. Football was my greatest passion, and in high school we made it to the state finals two years in a row. We lost my senior year, but not before we got the once-in-a-lifetime opportunity to play at Giants Stadium.

After high school I went to Montclair State University, which was about an hour away from Byram. I met a lot of amazing people there and even joined a fraternity. I graduated with degrees in computer science and mathematics. I was as active during my college years as I was during high school.

After college, I was hired by a software company in New York City. The company developed a proprietary user-sensing technology that provided training and statistical analysis for large-scale corporate applications such as PeopleSoft, IBM, SAP, and Kraft. I began as a solution developer and quickly advanced in responsibility, taking on managerial and technical sales responsibilities.

Within one year I was promoted to quality assurance manager and then to lead sales engineer. I was responsible for providing outside technical sales assistance to the sales team. I prepared and delivered corporate presentations, technical demonstrations, and product training to an international audience of prospective and pre-existing clients.

During the burst of the Internet Bubble in 2002, I left the company and established Hudson Horizons, a professional Web site design, development, and Internet marketing agency that provides innovative and quality services to businesses and corporations of all sizes. Over the last eight years, Hudson Horizons has transformed into a top-ranked company. Hudson Horizons has been ranked the number one Web development firm by a leading industry authority for two years and counting. We've also been listed in the Crain's New York BtoB Magazine Top Agency list. With our office headquartered in Saddle Brook, NJ, and our second office in Manhattan, NY, Hudson Horizons has turned into a nationally recognized agency.

At Hudson Horizons, I oversee the operations of the company. My main focus is to ensure that Hudson Horizons continues to expand and remains on top. I am responsible for managing the growth of Hudson Horizons on a daily basis. Since the Web industry is constantly changing, my team and I strive to keep Hudson Horizons ahead of the curve while continuing to produce innovative technology, and cutting edge services and solutions to our customers. In addition, I try to serve as a role model for my employees and aim to inspire my team through good work ethic, team-building events, and industry seminars.

I also believe in giving back to the community. I volunteer and make financial and other contributions to a number of charities, including Montel Williams MS Foundation, National MS Society, Big Brothers Big Sisters, Westside Infant and Teen Parent Program, Breast Cancer Prevention Institute, and the American Red Cross.

It was during my time at the software company in Manhattan that I was first diagnosed with MS, but I chose to deny my symptoms until shortly after beginning Hudson Horizons. During that time I was a very active person who took a proactive role in my life. The symptoms of MS could easily have stopped me in my tracks if I had let them, but I didn't.

Today, I am a very happily married man. My wife and I were married in 2009, and as of the time of this book's writing, I am proud to say that I am going to be a father; our first child is on the way. I am an entrepreneur, public speaker, and very active in my community. I am living a very happy, healthy, and successful life with MS, and I know that you can do the same. I may not have been given a choice in the cards I was dealt, but I was certainly given options in how to play them. I have elected to make certain that my MS does not rule my life. By making the right choices and changes every day, I have made sure that I am the one in control of my future.

CHAPTER 1

What Is MS?

Before we delve into my story, I feel that it is important to take a deeper look at Multiple Sclerosis. MS is a serious disease that can range from mild to severe. It is important for you to understand that I am not a doctor, but rather a patient who has worked hard to learn as much as I can about this disease in the hope that I could lessen its affect on my life.

I also want to clarify that I know the severity of my symptoms may not be the same as yours. Some people are able to live with MS for decades with only minimal symptoms, while others experience a sudden onset and are quickly thrown into a cycle of depression, worry, and medical struggles. Every case and every patient is different. My story is my experience. I hope that you can use my struggles and the knowledge and experience that came from them to help make yours easier.

Multiple Sclerosis is an autoimmune disease. Many of the most common medical conditions these days are autoimmune, including Crohn's disease, colitis, diabetes, and rheumatoid arthritis. In these diseases, the body's immune cells attack healthy, normal tissue as though it were a foreign invader. With MS, the immune cells attack the central nervous system along the brain and spinal cord.

As the immune system attacks the nervous system, inflammation develops. This damages the myelin sheath that protects the nerve cells. As this protective covering is damaged or destroyed, the nerve impulses slow greatly or even stop altogether.

MS is a progressive disease, which means that it will get worse over time. The rate at which the disease will progress is different from one person to the next and can be very slow or quite rapid. MS can develop and be diagnosed at any age, although it is most common for people to be diagnosed between the ages of twenty and forty. Studies show that women are more likely to be affected than men, and diagnostic rates are higher in the northern United States, southern Australia, and New Zealand.

The exact cause of Multiple Sclerosis is unknown. Scientists believe that the most likely causes are a genetic defect or perhaps a virus. Many believe that it is a combination of these two factors that results in the development and diagnosis of MS.

Symptoms and Complications

The symptoms of MS are incredibly varied, both in their type and severity. MS episodes, also known as flare-ups or relapses, can create symptoms virtually anywhere in the body. They may be triggered by diet, sun exposure, fever, stress, hot baths, or have no discernible cause at all. Symptoms can occur in almost any bodily system. Below you will find a listing of some of the most common symptoms of Multiple Sclerosis.

Muscle Symptoms

- Muscle spasms
- Numbness, burning, or tingling, especially in the arms and legs
- Weakness or tremors in the arms or legs
- Pain in the arms or legs
- Loss of balance
- Numbness or abnormal sensations anywhere in the body
- Problems moving the arms or legs
- Difficulty walking
- Difficulty making small movements
- Problems with coordination

Eye Symptoms

- Eye pain or discomfort
- Uncontrollable eye movement

- Double vision
- Vision loss (typically affecting only one eye at a time)

Bladder and Bowel Symptoms

- Strong urge to urinate
- Incontinence (urine leakage)
- Frequent need to urinate
- Difficulty starting urine stream
- Constipation
- Stool leakage

Sexual Problems

- Problems creating vaginal lubrication
- Erectile problems

Brain and Nerve Problems

- Slurred or hard to understand speech
- Trouble swallowing or chewing
- Difficulty reasoning
- Difficulty solving problems
- Sadness and depression
- Hearing loss
- Balance problems
- Dizziness
- Poor judgment
- Memory loss
- Decreased attention span

As MS progresses, fatigue also becomes a common issue. For many, the symptom is worse in the late afternoon. Fatigue can become very bothersome, as it grows more common and more severe.

Over time, complications can arise from MS. Not everyone will experience these complications. Their likelihood depends on the severity of the disease, lifestyle, treatment that the patient chooses, and a number of other factors. What follows are some potential complications of MS:

- Difficulty swallowing
- Depression
- Difficulty thinking
- Urinary tract infections
- Osteoporosis or bone thinning
- The need for catheterization
- A diminished ability to care for oneself
- Pressure sores

Testing and Diagnosing MS

Because there are many nervous system disorders whose symptoms may mimic or overlap those of MS, diagnosing the disease is largely a matter of ruling out other conditions.

MS is often suspected when there is a decreased function in more than one part of the nervous system on different occasions. For people with the form of MS known as relaps-ing-remitting, there is often a history of more than one episode (relapse) with a period in between in which few or no symptoms are present (remission).

There are a few exams and diagnostic tests that can be helpful in diagnosing MS. For example, a neurological exam can help locate an area of the body with reduced nerve function that presents a decreased sensation, decreased ability to move certain parts of the body, or abnormal nerve reflexes. An eye exam might also reveal problems with the eye, including rapid eye movements, decreased visual acuity, changes in movement, or abnor-mal responses by the pupil.

There are also a few diagnostic tests that can help iden-tify and diagnose MS. A spinal tap or lumbar puncture, for example, can allow for certain tests of the spinal fluid to help identify MS. An MRI of the spine and brain can help with diagnosis and also help track the progression of the disease. Nerve function tests can also help with both diag-nosis and progress charting of MS.

Treating MS

While the purpose of this book is to help you learn new ways to better treat your MS, there are also a number of treatments that are recommended by physicians. There is no known cure for MS, but there are many things you can do to help control symptoms and slow the progression of the disease. Following the advice of your physician is very important. The information learned in these pages is meant to help you change your lifestyle and to provide a supplement to medications and therapies offered by your doctor.

Pharmaceutical drug therapy is an essential element of MS treatment. There are specific medications that have been proven to help slow the progression of the disease. In this book, we will call these medications *ABC drugs*, a reference to the most common medications, which are Avonex, Betaseron, and Copaxone. Steroids may also be used in some patients to help reduce the overall severity of an MS attack. Medications are also frequently used to help reduce muscle spasms, urinary problems, depression, mood problems, and fatigue. While these medications often have side effects, their benefits typically make them advisable. Speaking with your doctor about these side effects can help you find ways to manage them; it's important to understand the drugs that might react differently with your body.

Medication is only one area of treatment when it comes to managing Multiple Sclerosis. Many patients find great benefit in physical, occupational, and speech therapy. Support groups offer a place for patients to come together to share both the physical and emotional effects of the disease on their own lives, and to help share ideas to lessen symptoms or make the disease easier to manage.

Exercise, rest, and proper nutrition are essential to reducing the severity and symptoms of MS. Learning relaxation techniques has also proven beneficial for many patients, and avoiding extreme temperatures, stress, and fatigue can help prevent relapses. Taking steps to avoid illness whenever possible can be very beneficial.

As the disease progresses, some MS patients find that they benefit from the use of assistive devices. This can include bed lifts, shower chairs, wheelchairs, and walkers. Don't hesitate to make changes to your household that can make movement safer and easier—those changes can prove extremely beneficial when symptoms are at their worst.

Prognosis

The outlook for patients with MS can be very hard to predict. Some people may experience a mild onset and a slow progression, while others experience a rapid onset and progression. However, there is a great deal of evidence that supports the fact that a healthy lifestyle, a prescribed medication regimen, and proper life changes can greatly improve the prognosis for MS patients, as it has done for me.

The majority of people living with MS are able to continue their lifestyles and jobs with minimal disturbance and disability for two decades or more. For many patients, life expectancy can be normal or close to it. Those diagnosed before the age of thirty, those with relapsing-remitting MS or occasional attacks, and those with limited forms of the disease have the best overall prognosis.

Determining the level of disability and the level of discomfort that will accompany MS is difficult. The frequency and severity of a relapse certainly plays a role, as well as the area of the nervous system that is affected by the attack. In between relapses, many people experience periods of normal function (remission), though over time, the amount of healing between episodes and the amount of restored function can diminish. Many patients find that as the disease progresses so does the need for assistive devices. With a strong support system and the right lifestyle changes, most patients are able to remain in their homes throughout the duration of the illness.

Summary

I hope this chapter gave you a clearer understanding of the medical definition, diagnosis, and treatment for MS. Keep in mind that every case is unique and symptoms, progression, and severity are different for every individual. It is this understanding of MS that will help you understand my story, the changes I have made, and how you can use these changes to help alter your story. This book is very much a tale of personal success, and I am hopeful that it will help you create your own success story.

MS has the power to destroy us mentally and physically if we allow it. You may not be able to cure the condition, but there is much you can do to change both your mind-set and your outcome. As we move forward, I hope that you will allow my experiences and my trials to help you overcome your symptoms and emotions so that you, too, can experience a healthier and happier life with Multiple Sclerosis.

CHAPTER 2

My Story

The story of my road to MS and my eventual ability to live a happy and fulfilling life with the disease has not been an easy one. There have been a lot of bumps along the way, and there have been both good times and bad. I feel that it is like this for any patient battling the disease. While my story is now a very happy one, it is important to know that there was a fight to make it to this point, and that if you are willing to work at it, you can be here, too.

The First Sign

The first time I noticed symptoms that started leading me to the diagnosis of MS, I was twenty-four years old. I had started noticing that the vision in my right eye was getting worse with each day that went by. This continued every day for about two weeks, and then, just as suddenly as it had appeared, it went away. Looking back now, I know that this should have been some sort of warning sign, but as strange as it was, I thought nothing of it. I felt fine otherwise, so I figured that whatever it was had simply run its course.

Later on the same year, 2002, I started noticing pain in my left eye. Soon, I started to lose vision. It began with slight pain but within a few days my whole eye socket started to feel as though someone was squeezing it with a wrench. It was unbearable. I couldn't move my eye at all, and over the next few days, the vision continued to worsen. Eventually, my vision became pixilated and looked as though everything was made up of giant dots. I couldn't figure out what was going on so I contacted my eye doctor for an appointment.

The eye doctor told me that everything looked normal. I tried to explain that this was not possible as my eye was in excruciating pain and everything was pixilated. He decided to send me to a specialist, who ended up telling me the same thing—there was no damage and my eye was fine. I wondered how that could possibly be. I was becoming frustrated and during the weeks and months that followed, the vision in my left eye became so pixilated that I nearly lost all vision. Worst of all, the pain never went away. I knew there had to be an answer out there.

Searching for a Solution

In 2003, I was referred to a neurologist at a university hospital in New Jersey. I explained my symptoms, and he immediately diagnosed me with optic neuritis. He explained that it is essentially an inflammation of the optic nerve that occurs suddenly. The inflammation can injure the insulation around each of the nerve fibers, causing the nerves themselves to swell. The swelling causes loss of vision, altered reaction to light, loss of color vision, and pain when moving the eye. That certainly sounded like what I was experiencing.

What scared me wasn't the diagnosis, but what the specialist said next. He told me that I needed an MRI of the brain to test for Multiple Sclerosis, as optic neuritis is often one of the first signs of the disease. I asked him what exactly Multiple Sclerosis was, and he explained the disease to me. It was absolutely terrifying to think, at the age of twenty-five, I could have a disabling disease that has no cure. There were so many questions running through my mind at that moment and in the days and weeks that followed.

Soon after that initial appointment I had an MRI of my brain. They found two lesions, called plaques, which are scars or scleroses within the central nervous system. Combined with the two exacerbations of optic neuritis I had experienced in 2002, it was enough to fulfill the diagnostic criteria for MS, which requires two separate episodes or relapses.

There I was, alone with the doctor, no friends or family around to support me, learning that I have Multiple Sclerosis. I couldn't help but wonder how I could have this disease and how this could happen to me at my age. Deep down I knew that the neurologist might be right, but my brain was trying to convince me there was no way this could be true; the problems with my vision were probably just a fluke, and I didn't have this disease.

The neurologist told me that there was a clinical drug trial taking place that was comparing two of the injectable ABC drugs used to treat MS. He believed that I was a perfect candidate for the trial, and while I would not know which drug I would be taking, it would potentially offer me great benefit. I thought about it a great deal and even spoke with my family about it, but I ended up passing on the trial. In fact, I ended up opting not to take any drugs whatsoever in that early period following my diagnosis.

Looking back on the decision not to try drug treatment for my MS in the early stages after my diagnosis, I realize now that more than anything, I was having a hard time admitting to myself that I had MS. Taking the medicine would mean admitting that I had the disease. I still believed that the doctors were wrong, and I didn't want to take a medication that could have potentially harmful side effects to treat a condition I wanted so badly to believe I didn't have.

The End of Denial

I would like to tell you that I quickly came to my senses and started properly treating my MS, but that is not what happened. It took me nearly two years to come to terms with the disease. I started doing research into MS beyond what I learned at doctor appointments. I researched what foods I should be eating and which I should be avoiding. I looked into vitamins and supplements, as well as natural and homeopathic treatments and solutions.

During this time, I also became very active in online forums where other MS patients would discuss what they were going through and what was working or not working for them. I wanted to find every solution I could that didn't involve taking the ABC injectable drugs. I still wanted so badly to avoid conventional medication.

While I now understand that the ABC drugs are an integral part of MS treatment, no matter how great your lifestyle and diet may be, I didn't realize that at the time. I recommend that all patients utilize online forums and research when learning about the disease and looking for solutions that can work for them. There is a real sense of community out there and there are some amazing people who will work to help ensure that you understand what is happening, what can happen, and that you can be okay. Learning how others are fighting the disease is very important to your ultimate success.

During these years, I was having nearly continuous bouts with optic neuritis. My vision would worsen, and my eyes would grow excruciatingly painful, then my vision would be restored and the pain would ease. Loss of color would come and go, and all of the other symptoms would appear and disappear. Despite this, I still chose to believe these symptoms were from the optic neuritis and not the MS, which the doctors said was causing it. I learned that the heat of the New Jersey summer really exacerbated my symptoms, and I would experience optic neuritis all three months during the summer. It was miserable, tiring, and incredibly hard to bear. It took a physical and emotional toll on me. It was the beginning of the end of my denial.

The Day That Changed My Life

One day in 2007, I was sitting at my desk using the computer at work. I began to feel nauseous and dizzy. I told my business partner that I was going to step outside for a bit of fresh air. I went out to sit in my car with the windows rolled down for a few minutes when suddenly I began violently vomiting. I felt extremely off balance and dizzy, and no matter what I did, I could not stop vomiting.

During this time, I started thinking that I was literally going to die. It terrified me. I should have called 911 and waited for an ambulance, but instead I decided to drive home. I phoned my girlfriend, who is now my wife, and asked her to call 911 to have the ambulance meet me at my house.

This of course, caused my girlfriend to panic. She began asking me what was wrong. I explained that I wasn't quite sure but that I was violently ill and needed her to call 911 right away so the ambulance would be there when I got home. The entire ride home felt as though I was driving drunk. In retrospect, I know that I should not have gotten behind the wheel. I was terrified and just wanted to get home.

Throughout the drive, I couldn't see a thing. My vision was incredibly blurry, and I had to drive with my door open so I could vomit every thirty seconds or so. That twenty-minute drive felt like it took an hour, and I truly believed that my life was coming to an end. I had never felt like that before, and it was the most frightening thing that has ever happened to me.

I made it to my house, and my girlfriend arrived shortly after I did. Within a few minutes, the ambulance arrived to pick me up. I vomited throughout the entire ride to the hospital. It was very surreal and strange, and all I could wonder was what could possibly be going on with me.

Once I was at the hospital, they ran a number of tests. I told the doctors that I had been diagnosed with MS, so they ordered a brain MRI to see if anything had changed since the last tests that were run in 2003. I even vomited in the MRI machine. It was absolutely horrible.

They told me that I was going to need to stay in the hospital overnight. That night turned into seven nights. During that time, I saw a number of specialists and doctors, all offering little result. That all changed when they brought in an ophthalmologist who took a look at my eyes and said, "You have nystagmus."

I asked the ophthalmologist what exactly nystagmus was, and she explained that it is a medical condition that presents with involuntary shaking and movement of the eyes. It causes a loss of balance and equilibrium and problems with blurring vision. She said that my left eye was fluttering side to side, while the right was moving up and down. They were moving so rapidly that they looked like the wings of a hummingbird in flight.

Experiencing vision problems and vomiting was bad enough on its own, but to top it all off, I was no longer able to walk. The moment I stood up, I fell over to the left. I had been walking for almost thirty years, and all of a sudden I couldn't take a single step without falling to the ground. The doctors told me it would take some time for everything to return to normal, and I learned that it would take some time for the realization that I truly had MS to sink in as well. It seemed surreal that these things were really happening to me.

Once I had a clear diagnosis (and one that was definitely related to the MS), the hospital put me on an IV steroid treatment. Steroids are used to help reduce the severity and duration of exacerbations or relapses. After my seven days in the hospital, the nystagmus was finally beginning to subside. I was allowed to go home when I was able to walk with only the assistance of a cane. Once home, I spent a few days resting, and after a few weeks, I started to feel normal again.

When the MRI results came in, they were shocking. The two brain lesions that were on the MRI I had in 2003 had now become seven, and one of the lesions was located directly on my brain stem. The brain stem essentially controls the entire body, including the heart, and it is connected to the spinal cord. This caused me to sit up and take notice of what was going on.

Since the nystagmus was an exacerbation or flare-up of the MS and because I'd experienced a more than sixfold increase in the number of lesions on my brain, the neurologist I saw while in the hospital took the time to stress to me how important it was to immediately go on one of the ABC injectable drugs. While these drugs cannot cure MS, they could help slow the progression of the disease. For once, I was willing to listen.

For Better and Worse: Making Life-Altering Changes

After going through this suffering, it was no longer possible for me to deny that I had MS. Instead, I needed to look myself in the mirror and face the condition head on. While this may sound easy, it was anything but. I realized that if I didn't want this disease to take over my life or to reduce the quality and quantity of it, I had no choice.

It was at this time that I started to become incredibly serious about changing my life, including diet, exercise, supplements, vitamins, and ultimately my mindset. All these things will be discussed in-depth later on in this book, but for now it is important to realize that that week of my life and the diagnoses that followed made all the difference in my attitude and determination to change.

With the help and support of my family, I decided to set out in search of a top neurologist. There was no way to deny that the MS had gotten worse. I finally realized that it was crucial I start taking one of the ABC injectable drugs and that I start seeing a neurologist on a regular basis.

One of my family members brought to my attention a magazine article about the top neurologists in New Jersey, and I used it to choose a neurologist who seemed right for my case. At our first meeting, he immediately started me on one of the ABC injectable drugs most commonly used for treating MS. I have chosen not to name it because each individual's experience (side effects and benefits) with a drug is unique and because that drug may well be the one that helps make a life-altering difference for someone else.

I was on that drug for two years, and during that time I could not get past the horrible side effects. After each injection, I would suffer terrible flu-like symptoms for about fifteen hours. I don't just mean the sniffles, either. I mean muscle aches, pain, chills, a fever—the whole nine yards. I ended up taking over-the-counter flu medicine with every injection though it did little to alleviate my symptoms.

Of course, the flu symptoms were only the beginning. Over time, I started to become irritable and depressed. The depression only seemed to deepen over time, and eventually I reached a point where I no longer wanted to live. I wasn't going to act on those impulses, but I truly thought about suicide every day.

I told my fiancée that I didn't want to take the medication anymore because I could no longer handle the depression and suicidal thoughts. It was turning me into a person who was always sick, depressed, and angry. Worse still, I often felt as though I couldn't live with the disease anymore and wanted to die.

When I finally decided to tell my doctor about the suicidal thoughts I had been having, he immediately told me that I needed to come off of the drug. He said that we could try something different. We discussed all my options and settled on another ABC injectable drug.

The new drug needed to be injected daily but used a smaller needle. Most importantly, with the new drug, I had few to no side effects at all. This took precedence over needle size or injection frequency. I needed my life back. I needed to feel like myself again. There was simply no way I could keep living with the side effects of the first drug any longer. I was very excited at the prospect of starting a new treatment and a new regimen.

The Big Switch

Since I was starting on a new medication, my doctor wanted me to get an MRI to see how things had changed in the last two years. My doctor and I were both quite pleased to see that all seven lesions had decreased in both size and activity. They were not nearly as bright as they were on my previous MRI, which meant that the medication I had been taking, despite its horrible effects on my personality and mood, had definitely been working to slow the progression of the MS.

There is no doubt in my mind that my lifestyle changes played a large role in this improvement, but the effects of the drug could not be denied. While the lesions didn't disappear, they became smaller and less active and that was cause for celebration. It meant that this wasn't hopeless any longer.

Once I started the new drug, all sorts of worries crept in. Was changing to a new drug really the right move, considering the benefit that my disease saw from the first drug? Should I have just learned to deal with the side effects of the original medication? Would this change cause a setback or force my disease to get as bad as it once was?

Shortly after I started taking the new medication, I started to experience numbness in my entire body. It started in my legs, moved up into my groin, spread to my hands and my arms, and eventually to my neck and face. It was frightening, especially the numbness in my groin. There was no sensation when I touched my skin, and that freaked me out. The muscles themselves were not numb, but my skin had become numb to the touch.

My doctor prescribed oral steroids that started to ease the numbness over time, but I lived with almost total numbness for several weeks. It took about two months for the numbness to go away. My doctor thinks it may be the result of the old medication leaving my system while the new medication still needed time to kick in.

Life Today

I have been on the new drug for some time now, and I am careful to take it as prescribed. I also strive to have the healthiest lifestyle possible. I am so much happier than I was years ago. My depression is gone, I have no side effects, and I have not had any more exacerbations or relapses. Also, I haven't experienced any numbness—anywhere.

It's hard to believe that just a few years ago I was at complete rock bottom, convinced I didn't want to and couldn't live with this disease anymore. I think back on that time, on that guy, and just can't believe he was me. The new medication and my new lifestyle changed everything.

CHAPTER 3

Conventional Medicine

As I mentioned in the last chapter when I was first diagnosed, and in the few years that followed, I was very hesitant to try conventional medicine. At first, I was simply in denial that I had this disease, and then I started to convince myself I could manage it without the use of drugs. While a healthy and balanced lifestyle made a huge difference for me, I now know that I should have considered conventional medicine from the start.

I have no doubt that supplements and healthy living are essential to a healthy and happy life with MS, but it is also my belief that everyone with MS should be on some form of conventional drug therapy as well. There are simply too many benefits from these drugs for them to be ignored, especially in light of their potential to slow the progression of the disease.

What Conventional Medicine Offers

Conventional medicinal treatment for MS means using disease-modifying drugs. The most common options for this are the ABC drugs. There are a number of choices in terms of injectable drugs, ranging from shots that must be injected daily to those that are injected only every four weeks. The FDA has approved an oral disease-modifying drug for MS, but it is not necessarily the right choice for everyone. Many people will continue to find injectable drugs to offer the most benefit.

Taking disease-modifying drugs is incredibly important when it comes to treating Multiple Sclerosis. These drugs can help reduce both the frequency and severity of relapses or flare-ups, and, as noted earlier, they appear to slow down the rate at which patients become disabled by the disease. They also help reduce the accumulation of lesions on the brain and spinal cord, as well as the activity that occurs within the lesions. These statements are based on MRI examinations of patients who are using the drugs as indicated.

While no drug can cure MS, disease-modifying medications can slow the progression of the disease and make its effects more manageable. There are currently eight disease-modifying drugs that have been approved by the FDA for the treatment of relapsing forms of MS, including one that is also approved for secondary-progressive MS.

26

If you have been diagnosed with MS, it is crucial that you speak with a qualified neurologist about getting started on a disease-modifying drug therapy. Speak openly and honestly about your lifestyle and habits. Ask your doctor about the potential risks, benefits, and side effects of each medication. The course of your disease and your lifestyle will play a large role in determining what medication your doctor believes is right for you.

It's important to understand that every MS patient's body will react differently to the various medications, and your body may respond differently. If the first medication you try isn't the one for you, don't give up on drug therapy. These medications can offer years of reduced symptoms and can help slow the progression of the disease, especially when combined with the right lifestyle changes.

Doing your own research on these medications will allow you to learn what to expect and can encourage you to speak openly with your doctor about what might be the best course of action for you. Take an active approach to your treatment and health care. You know your body better than anyone, and you can work with your doctor to find the solution that is most likely to work for you.

Disease-Modifying Drugs

When investigating the right course of drug therapy for you, it is essential to look at all the viable drugs. The list below offers the eight disease-modifying drugs currently available in alphabetical order. You can read how the drug is taken, at what frequency, and why it is often prescribed. The most common side effects and any rare reactions that patients should watch for are also discussed.

This list is not intended to be a definitive method for choosing a drug therapy. It's purpose is to educate you about these drugs and help you determine the drugs on which you may want to focus in your research and when speaking with your health care professional.

Avonex

This drug is an injectable medication that is given once per week in the muscle. It is primarily used for relapsing forms of MS to help slow the rate of disability and to reduce the frequency of exacerbations. It is used with patients who have experienced their first clinical episode and who have MRI features that are consistent with a diagnosis of MS. Common side effects include flu-like symptoms after the injection, which often lessen over time. Rare but possible symptoms to watch out for include depression, liver abnormalities, allergic reactions, and heart problems.

Betaseron

This injectable is given under the skin every other day and is, like Avonex, primarily used for relapsing forms of MS to help slow the rate of disability and reduce exacerbation frequency. It is also used for patients who have experienced a first clinical episode and have MRI features that are consistent with MS. Common side effects are flu-like symptoms, which often lessen over time, and injection-site reactions that in about 5 percent of cases need medical attention. Rare but possible side effects to watch for include allergic reaction, liver abnormalities, low white-blood-cell counts, and depression.

Copaxone

Copaxone is a daily injectable that is given under the skin. This drug is also given for relapsing-remitting MS to help reduce the number of clinical exacerbations. It is intended for patients who have experienced a first clinical episode and have MRI features consistent with MS. Common side effects include injection-site reactions. Rare side effects include chest pain and narrowing of blood vessels. It is also possible to experience a reaction including chest pain, flushing, shortness of breath, anxiety, and palpitations shortly after injections. This reaction lasts less than thirty minutes, resolves without treatment, and has no lasting effects.

Extavia

Extavia is injected under the skin (subcutaneously) every other day. This drug is used for treating relapsing forms of MS to help reduce the frequency of exacerbations and is used in patients who have had a first clinical episode and who have MRI features consistent with a diagnosis of Multiple Sclerosis. Common side effects include flu-like symptoms after injection that frequently lessen over time, as well as injection-site reactions that require medical attention about 5 percent of the time. Less common effects to look out for include allergic reactions, low white-blood-cell counts, liver abnormalities, and depression.

Gilenya

Gilenya is a daily oral capsule. It is prescribed to treat relapsing forms of MS and to reduce the frequency of exacerbations and to delay the accumulation of physical disability. Common side effects include headache, diarrhea, fever, liver enzyme elevations, cough, and back pain. Less common reactions include infection, swelling of the eye, and a slowed heart rate after the first dose.

Novantrone

This drug, which is also available in generic form, is given intravenously four times per year in a medical facility. A patient may not receive more than eight to twelve doses of this drug in his or her lifetime; the drug is atypically given over a period of two to three years. The drug is given for worsening relapsing-remitting MS, progressive-relapsing MS, and secondary progressive MS. It helps reduce neurologic disability, as well as the frequency of clinical exacerbations. Common side effects include blue-green urine in the twenty-four hours following administration of the drug, nausea, hair thinning, bladder infections, mouth sores, and bone-marrow suppression, which is hallmarked by fatigue, low blood-cell counts, and bruising. Patients taking this drug must also be monitored for serious heart and liver damage.

Rebif

This drug is injected subcutaneously three times weekly. It is used to treat relapsing forms of MS to help reduce the frequency of clinical exacerbations and can also help delay the accumulation of physical disability. Common side effects include flu-like symptoms following injection, as well as injection-site reactions. Less common symptoms to look for include depression, allergic reaction, low red- or white-blood-cell counts, and liver abnormalities.

Tysabri

This drug is given intravenously every four weeks in a registered infusion facility. It is used only when no other disease modifying medications are being used and is designed to treat relapsing forms of MS to delay the accumulation of physical disability and to reduce the frequency of exacerbations. It is primarily used for patients who cannot tolerate other disease-modifying drugs or who have an inadequate response to those drugs. Common side effects include headache, fatigue, depression, lower respiratory tract infections, urinary tract infections, chest discomfort, and joint pain. Less common effects include allergic reactions within two hours of infusion (hallmarked by fever, rash, dizziness, trouble breathing, chest pain, nausea, and itching), as well as liver abnormalities. This drug can also increase the risk for a rare and often fatal brain disease called progressive multifocal leukoencephalopathy (PML) for which your physician will monitor you closely.

About Side Effects

Side effects are possible with any medication that you take, whether it is an over-the-counter pain reliever or a disease-modifying drug. With drugs for MS, however, it is absolutely essential that you inform your doctor of any and all side effects you experience. Depending on the severity of the effects, it is also important to realize that you may need to learn to live with them in order to help keep the disease under control. There are medications out there that can help lessen certain side effects. Your doctor will work with you to help ensure that your effects are as manageable as possible.

You will find that in many cases side effects, such as flu-like symptoms, can be managed. In my case, it was not possible to manage my symptoms or my depression, as these continued to worsen over time. However, I have spoken to other MS patients whose flu-like symptoms actually decreased as time went on. It's important to remember that many side effects may lessen in severity the longer you are on a specific medication. Speak with your doctor about the side effects you are experiencing from any drug you are taking. Ensure that you inform your physician of any other medications and supplements that you are on to help prevent interactions. Many drugs require periodic blood tests to check for liver damage, problems in your blood cell counts, and iron levels.

Conventional Therapy Is Important

While side effects are certainly undesirable, every drug on this list has been shown to help reduce the frequency of relapses and the development of new lesions on the brain and spinal cord. In addition to lessening symptoms and lesion formation, these drugs can also help prevent brain atrophy or shrinkage, which happens when the myelin nerve sheath is destroyed by a lesion. Limiting lesion formation and growth is essential to reducing the chances of permanent disability in the future. Taking these drugs as early as possible after diagnosis and taking them as prescribed or indicated is crucial.

The medication that is right for you will depend on the severity of your disease, your lifestyle, and how you react to the medication. Speaking openly and honestly with your doctor about your lifestyle, symptoms, and side effects is the best way to find the right drug for you. Conventional drug therapy can be immeasurably beneficial in the fight against MS.

The Bottom Line

Conventional drug therapy is an essential part of MS treatment, but it is only one piece of the puzzle. For me, the best way to learn how to manage my MS was to search through all of the resources that were available to me online. I knew that in addition to medication, I needed to look into alternative medicine, diet, exercise, vitamins, and supplements. When combined with drug therapy, these nutritional and lifestyle changes have proven to be incredibly important. In the next few chapters, we will look at the lifestyle changes I made and how those helped, in conjunction with the medications I was taken, to manage my MS. We will see how, when used together, they helped to greatly slow the progression of the disease within my body, to the point where I believe I have conquered this disease.

CHAPTER 4

Things Doctors Don't Tell You

When you are first diagnosed with MS, you are likely to have a lot of questions. You will want to know what the disease is, how it is treated, the prognosis for the average patient, and much more. These are all questions that your physician will work to answer for you. Most physicians will be very patient in explaining the disease, how it progresses, and what you can most likely expect in terms of symptoms and relapses.

With that said, there is also a lot that most doctors won't tell you. Most doctors will only discuss conventional treatments for MS, such as drug therapy. This is primarily because they are only able to offer FDA approved treatment instructions because of the threat of lawsuits that comes when offering information on nonconventional therapies. It also means that there are a large number of details and a great deal of potentially helpful information that is left out. Doctors are taught to believe in drug therapy and conventional treatment methods. While these drug therapies do go a long way in treating MS, I believe they are only part of the solution.

In the years following my diagnosis, I have done a great deal of research. I have looked into alternative therapies and remedies, and believe that these have played a large role in my progress. I believe that these things have helped to slow the progression of my disease. They have helped keep the number of new lesions low and helped reduce the activity of my existing lesions. I also believe that my combination of conventional and alternative therapy has brought me as close as possible to a cure for my MS.

Since being diagnosed, I have experimented with a number of different diets, exercise regimens, supplements, vitamins, and herbs. I have worked hard to understand the effects of each on my body and my disease; I also have worked to understand how the regimens I ultimately chose have affected my progress. I believe that these things have worked alongside the drugs to help repair and improve the parts of my body that have been damaged by MS.

There are a number of things that doctors don't tell MS patients, including certain links between diet and lower incidence rates. For example, Omega 3 oils are shown to be essential for the formation of the myelin sheath that protects nerves, but because these oils are typically taken as non-FDA regulated supplements, many doctors do not tell patients about this link.

Another thing that is often overlooked or mentioned only briefly is the link between stress and MS exacerbations. Numerous studies show that even everyday stress can make symptoms more severe or even cause relapses. Diet and exercise can help alleviate stress, as can certain other lifestyle changes and treatments. Learning about this link can offer great benefit to patients, yet it is one that is rarely addressed by physicians and health care professionals.

The discovery of things like the effect of stress led me to do much research of my own when it came to this disease. I recommend that other patients do the same. Look into the studies, research the treatments, and join the online communities. There are people all over the world who are battling MS, and it is only when you look at both the conventional and alternative treatments that you can truly help slow or stop the progression of the disease in your body.

CHAPTER 5

Diet and You

When it comes to diets, the possibilities are nearly limitless. If you Google *diet plans*, you will find thousands of diet suggestions for almost any symptom, disease, or issue. The same is true for MS. The fact of the matter is that diet plays an essential role in helping to prevent exacerbations and symptoms of this disease.

It is important for me to make the distinction that I am neither a registered dietician nor a nutritionist. However, I have spent countless hours researching the various diets that are suggested for MS. In this chapter, I will look at many of the diets out there that are often recommended for MS patients, including the diet I have chosen for myself.

The Swank Diet

One of the most popular diet plans for people with MS is the Swank Diet. While this is not the diet that I personally use, there are many MS patients who have had great success with it. The Swank Diet was formulated after a fifty-year period of research that followed hundreds of patients.

Sixty years ago, Dr. Roy Swank first found that a low-fat diet could help people with MS live healthier and happier lives. Since then, he has recommended the diet to many and has done a great deal of research on the effects of certain foods on MS. In fact, many of the earliest patients who followed the Swank Diet are still ambulatory and independent almost a half a century later.

The Swank Diet is not just about eating low-fat foods. It also means choosing foods that are low in saturated fats, polyunsaturated oils, and red and fatty meats. The diet is high in grains, fruits, and vegetables, and has helped many people alleviate some of the most chronic symptoms of MS. Much of the Swank Diet is based on the realization that MS rates and disease rates, as a whole, have increased as people move toward diets that are higher in processed and fatty foods.

The Swank MS Foundation advocates starting the diet as soon as possible after diagnosis and combining it with rest, reduced stress, exercise, and a positive attitude. The diet means using only fat-free or nonfat dairy products, using whole grains and bread products, abstaining from commercially prepared foods, avoiding mayonnaise and most caffeine, limiting alcohol, and eating at least two fruits daily. Nuts are also recommended, as well as vegetables, turkey, shellfish, and white fish. Pork and red meat are not allowed in the first year on the Swank Diet, and there are many vitamin and supplement recommendations that should be taken in order to properly adhere to the regimen.

There are a vast number of rules in the Swank Diet, and all must be adhered to in order for the full benefit to be achieved. The Swank MS Foundation believes that while learning this new lifestyle is a challenge, it is a far smaller challenge than living with a disability. Treating your MS is about finding the option that is right for you, and the Swank Diet is one to consider.

Low-Sugar Diets

A low-sugar diet is also a common choice for people with MS. There is certainly scientific backing for this diet, as studies by the UK Allergy and Nutrition Center show the diagnostic incidence of MS is considerably higher in parts of the world that consume the most sugar. It is important to note that the Mayo Clinic and similar institutions do not specifically recommend a low-sugar diet but do recommend a balanced diet that is low in sugar.

The goal of the low-sugar diet is to eliminate high-sugar foods because they are believed to exacerbate symptoms. This means always checking the ingredients list on labels for sugar, corn syrup, high fructose corn syrup, maltodextrin, sucrose, dextrose, and sorbitol. The key is to replace these foods with fruits, vegetables, and lean proteins. This diet can be a good way to learn if sugar-laden foods exacerbate your condition since if they do, eliminating them for a prolonged period of time would result in a decrease in symptom severity.

Gluten-Free Diet

The gluten free diet is most commonly associated with celiac disease, another autoimmune condition. In fact, it is a condition that is often misdiagnosed as MS and vice versa because the symptoms of each can be so broad. Studies show that eliminating gluten can be helpful in controlling and even reducing MS symptoms.

Gluten is a protein that is found in wheat, barley, rye, millet, and oats. It is also a binding agent used in the production of many types of bread and pasta that helps keep the dough together. It is found in many common products including chips, beer, and crackers.

An excellent way to determine if the gluten-free diet is a good choice for you is to try a two-week elimination approach. This means avoiding all foods containing gluten for a full two weeks and then reintroducing the ingredient on the fifteenth day. For many patients, this two-week period is marked by a reduction in symptoms, while the reintroduction of gluten on the fifteenth day can present with anything from intestinal distress, sore muscles, emotional imbalance, anxiety, migraine, fatigue, and stomach upset. If this happens for you, then the gluten-free diet will offer you great benefit.

I have chosen to completely eliminate gluten from my diet. I become bloated and experience intestinal distress when I eat food that contains gluten. I experience a sense of nervousness and anxiety in my chest that makes my heart feel like it is shutting down. I know that gluten is very bad for my body, and my research has helped me learn that gluten can actually cause a number of problems and even autoimmune conditions in people with MS.

If you experience any of the symptoms of gluten intolerance such as joint pain, stomach upset, bloating, muscle aches, nervousness, fatigue, anxiety, mood swings, or inflammation after eating products containing gluten, you may wish to speak with your doctor. There are tests available that can help check you for gluten sensitivity. If you are gluten intolerant, eliminating it from your diet will make a significant difference. You will find that there are actually a number of gluten-free versions of your favorite foods, including bread, pastas, beer, pizza, snacks, and much more now available in your neighborhood grocery store.

A Trigger-Free Diet

Another common change that people make when adopting the gluten-free diet is to eliminate legumes and dairy products from their diet. Studies show that both of these ingredients are common triggers for MS, just like gluten. These foods are common allergens, and legumes and wheat both contain substances known as lectins, which are very hard to digest and can even be toxic. It is believed that these cells can pass through into the bloodstream activating immune cells and nerve cells and wreaking havoc on the body.

While legumes are not triggers for everyone, for many people eliminating them from the diet can help stop current symptoms and keep new ones from developing. A great deal of creating an MS diet is about learning which foods trigger symptoms for you. For many people, this can be wheat, gluten, dairy, sugar, or legumes. The trigger-free diet is largely about eliminating foods to which people commonly exhibit sensitivities. For those who do not wish to undergo sensitivity testing or who only exhibit sensitivities during certain times, it can be the easiest way to eliminate potential triggers.

These triggers, along with fats and sugars, can cause symptoms to become exacerbated. When combined with stress, fatigue, health problems, or a poor exercise regimen, they can cause the symptoms to become almost unbearable. Eliminating trigger foods can prove challenging, especially for people who have enjoyed them for decades. The amount of relief that this can provide can make the change highly worthwhile.

The Best-Bet Diet

Because there are so many potential triggers for MS symptoms when it comes to diet, a diet has been created that eliminates all of the common trigger foods and ingredients. This is known as the Best-Bet Diet and it is recommended for many MS patients. Many believe that it can be effective in helping to slow the progression of MS.

While elimination tests can often help you figure out trigger foods, sensitivity may also be related to the level of stress and fatigue you are feeling at the time. The Best-Bet Diet eliminates all of the trigger foods, helping to ensure that your diet does not trigger symptoms for you.

With the Best-Bet Diet, patients eliminate all dairy, gluten, and legumes. They avoid eggs and yeast or only eat them in moderation. They also avoid margarine, processed sugar, and any foods identified as allergenic by ELISA tests. Saturated fats are limited to fifteen grams or less per day. Like other MS diets, the Best-Bet Diet is intended to be used in conjunction with changes in lifestyle, stress, and exercise.

The Best-Bet Diet is one I have chosen for myself; I have followed it for many years now and have seen great benefit from being on this diet. I urge everyone to at least look into the Best-Bet Diet, and see if it's right for you.

Turmeric

While not a specific diet, there is much anecdotal and scientific evidence that shows that turmeric can offer benefit for patients with MS. Turmeric is a natural anti-inflammatory agent. Studies show that it can be as effective as many major anti-inflammatory drugs but without the risk of side effects. It is also a very inexpensive additive that can offer huge benefits in terms of relief from the symptoms of Multiple Sclerosis.

I put a teaspoon of turmeric on many of my dinnertime meals. It has many health benefits to the body and also shown to help slow the progression of MS in mice. While it can have a bitter and earthy flavor, it makes a great complement to many dishes. For those who simply do not care for the taste, turmeric is also available in supplement form.

Yerba Mate

Yerba mate is a plant whose leaves are used in tea form, similar to green tea, and provides a natural source of energy. In fact, yerba mate has almost all of the same ingredients as green tea, as well as a number of other very powerful antioxidants. I drink four cups of yerba mate daily and highly recommend it to others. It not only makes me feel focused and mentally energetic, but also it gives me the stamina I need all day long without affecting my sleep.

This is something that coffee has never managed to do for me.

Dark Leafy Greens

While looking for natural anti-inflammatory agents, it is important to include dark leafy greens into your diet. These include kale, chard, broccoli rabe, and collard and mustard greens. Not only do these veggies contain incredible anti-inflammatory properties, but they are also rich in vitamins A, C, E, and K. These greens are also shown to help lower blood pressure and cholesterol, promote better GI function and eyesight, reduce your risk of heart disease, and even help lower your risk of certain types of cancer. It is recommended to eat at least one serving of organic dark leafy greens a day.

Fruits and Vegetables

Studies also show that fruit and vegetables can be very beneficial for people who have Multiple Sclerosis. While fruits and veggies are recommended for everyone as part of a healthy diet, they are essential for providing high levels of fiber, digestive support, and energy in people with MS. Fruits such as berries, apples, pears, and pomegranates and vegetables such as broccoli, carrots, cabbage, red beets, and tomatoes are packed with vitamins, nutrients, antioxidant properties, and offer excellent support for the digestive system. Eating two to three servings a day of both organic fruits and vegetables is highly recommended.

Pineapple

This tasty tropical fruit is high in the enzyme bromelain and the antioxidant vitamin C, both of which play a key role in the body's healing process. Bromelain is a natural anti-inflammatory that has many health benefits and promotes healing.

Bromelain also plays an active role in digestion. Studies have shown that the bromelain contained in fresh pineapple can relieve indigestion. The enzyme breaks down the amino acid bonds in protein, which promotes healthy digestion. Also, because of the high vitamin C content, pineapple helps the body fight off bacteria and other toxins that may harm the body.

Adding pineapple to your diet is a natural way to enhance your body's healing process and promote overall good health. It's a quick, easy, and tasty snack to add to your diet. Simply slice the pineapple or blend it into a drink or smoothie. Include the core, as the core is very high in bromelain.

Heart-Healthy Fats: The Mediterranean Diet

Another common diet choice for people with MS is the Mediterranean Diet. This diet consists of heart-healthy fats and a low-stress lifestyle. While the Mediterranean Diet grew out of the poverty that affected people in that region, studies showed that the diet led them to become among the healthiest people in the world when it came to certain diseases and health conditions.

The Mediterranean Diet consists of numerous nuts as well as taking in a great deal of Omega 3 fatty acids, which can be found in fish, especially those that are oily like salmon. A Mediterranean Diet also consists of a high consumption of extra virgin olive oil, coconut oil, vegetables, fruits, red wine, tomatoes, and goat-based cheese products. Adhering to this diet in conjunction with a healthy lifestyle is shown to be incredibly beneficial to people suffering from MS.

I have found the Mediterranean Diet mixed with the Best-Bet Diet had the best affect on my overall health. I have chosen to follow these two diets to help manage my MS and provide me with an overall healthy lifestyle.

The Organic Diet

There is a lot of attention surrounding organic foods these days and with good reason. Most of the foods you buy at the grocery store, including meats, vegetables, and fruits, are so laden with chemicals and hormones that they can lead to a number of health issues. Many of these chemicals even reduce the nutritional value of these foods. Eating organic fruits, vegetables, poultry, eggs, meats, and more can be incredibly beneficial. While not all restaurants offer organic selections, you should strive to eat them whenever possible.

Avoiding pesticides by eating organic can be incredibly beneficial to your MS. Pesticides leftover in vegetables and fruits can cause a number of health issues, including nervous system damage and even certain kinds of cancer. Antibiotics are often found in meats, as they are given to many animals that allow them to eat cheap foods that their bodies could not otherwise tolerate. Many doctors believe that this antibiotic exposure is at least partially responsible for the resistant nature of many illnesses to modern antibiotics. Avoiding milk and meat products that have been treated with hormones is equally important because the effects of the hormones can linger in the body.

A great idea is to look for products with labels such as USDA organic that let you know they are certified organic and safer for consumption than their conventional counterparts. Terms such as *free range* or *cage free*, *no added hormones*, and *no pesticides or antibiotics* are all important things to look for on product labels. The more organic foods you include in your diet, the less risk of unwanted effects from chemicals hidden in your food.

What Works for Me

The Best-Bet Diet has proven to be the most beneficial for me. I completely eliminate dairy and gluten. I minimize my sugar intake, being conscious of all product labels. I also enjoy a Mediterranean Diet that is high in Omega 3 fish oils, nuts, healthy fats, and that is comprised of organic foods whenever possible. This has helped to greatly improve the overall health and well being of my body, and I believe it to be one of the primary reasons why I am living symptom free with my MS.

I chose my diet based largely on the research that I have done, but also by experimenting to learn what my body tolerated best and what felt right for me. I have tried numerous options in terms of food elimination and have worked hard to find a diet that offers the improvements I seek but doesn't cause harm to my body. Finding the best diet can be difficult, time consuming, and even stressful, but it is absolutely time well spent when you consider the benefits for your overall health and happiness.

What Doesn't Work for Me

Just as there are certain things that I strive to put into my body to help reduce symptoms of MS, there are many things that I absolutely avoid as I strive to maintain as natural a diet as possible. In addition to foods laden with chemicals and hormones, the following ingredients and foods are those I strive to avoid at all costs.

Hydrogenated or Partially Hydrogenated Oils

These oils are very high in trans-fats. They have a number of adverse effects on health, including the fact that they cause you to eat more while slowing your metabolism. These oils raise blood pressure and cholesterol, damage arteries, and decrease circulation of the blood in the brain, which can worsen many physical health conditions, including MS. Hydrogenated oils are found in many snacks, fried foods, and packaged foods. Be sure to look at the food labels are these oils are found in many products in your average grocery store.

High Fructose Corn Syrup and High-Sugar Foods

High Fructose Corn Syrup (HFCS) is a highly purified blend of sugars, fructose, and glucose that is derived from corn. Because the fructose in HFCS is part of a man-made blend, as opposed to the natural compound of sugars found in fruit, the body metabolizes it very differently from other sugars. There are many reasons why doctors advise patients, even healthy ones, to avoid high-sugar diets. They can cause weight gain, dental problems, decreased nutrition, and increased triglycerides. They can also increase your risk of suffering a heart attack. I completely eliminated HFCS and other foods high in sugar from my diet altogether.

Aspartame

In recent years, there was a major health scare about the link between aspartame and MS. It has been reported by many that the ingredient actually increases the risk of getting MS. While there is some debate over the truth to this argument, there is evidence that the excitotoxins in aspartame can cause prolonged worsening of MS lesions. Because of this and because of many other unfavorable side effects, including headaches and an increased risk of certain cancers, aspartame is one ingredient I never allow into my diet.

Fried Foods

Fried foods have been totally eliminated from my diet. These foods are unhealthy just for their fat content alone, but when you realize that these foods are actually fried in hydrogenated oils, it becomes obvious just how bad they can be. Fried foods also contain acrylamide, which is a neurotoxin that can damage the central nervous system, which is already compromised in people with MS.

Coffee

I have found that one of the best decisions for me was to give up coffee. Every time I drink it, I feel very ill. My heart begins to flutter, and I get nauseous. My research has shown that high amounts of coffee may be detrimental for people with MS, so I elected to cut it from my diet and replace it with yerba mate.

The Bottom Line

The diet that works best for you may not be the same diet that works best for me. Learning what triggers or exacerbates your symptoms is a process of trial and error. Many physicians will recommend ELISA tests to help determine food sensitivities that may act as triggers for you. The Best-Bet Diet can also be helpful in avoiding foods that may produce symptoms. The road to the right diet for you will be different than mine, but I hope that my experience can help you see that there is a diet out there that can offer you significant improvement to your MS symptoms.

CHAPTER 6

Vitamins and Supplements

Natural medicine has been in existence for as long as humans have been on earth. Since ancient times, humans have studied the ways that various plants react with the body to help offer health benefits. Still today, we all know the link between vitamins, supplements, and better health. There are many vitamin supplements that can help reduce the symptoms and exacerbations associated with MS. It is my belief that the right combination of vitamins and supplements, in conjunction with a healthy lifestyle, diet, exercise, and conventional drug therapy can actually help to potentially eliminate the disease.

I have spent a great deal of time researching various vitamins and supplements in order to determine the regimen that I felt would offer my body the most benefit. I am now living completely free of MS symptoms, and I believe that the vitamin regimen I have chosen is largely responsible for this. In this chapter, we will look at the various supplements I take, the dosages I have chosen, and the benefits that they offer for people with MS. We will also look at herbal remedies that are touted for MS, including those that are not part of my own personal regimen.

Multivitamins

It is recommended that virtually everyone take a multivitamin. Most modern diets are incredibly nutrient deficient, especially for people who eat canned, processed, packaged, or commercially prepared foods. I choose a multivitamin that contains 100 percent or more of most major vitamins and nutrients, as well as minerals and herbal blends. In addition to helping with specifically MS-related symptoms, it helps improve the overall health and function of the body, which reduces stress, makes exercise more effective, and contributes to a stronger immune system.

Vitamin D3

I take 12,000 IU of vitamin D3 every day. This is roughly 3,000 percent of the daily value recommended by the FDA. Studies show that areas of the world where the diet is rich in D3, experience significantly lower incidence rates of MS. Taking a D3 supplement can help to dramatically reduce the relapse rate for MS patients.

Vitamin D is a natural immune system regulator that also helps control the metabolism of calcium. Studies show that people taking high doses of the vitamin can cut their chances of relapse by more than 41 percent. This is certainly a very significant number, especially when considering that this reduction can be found in the form of a vitamin naturally occurring in fish and from our body's manufacturing of sunlight. Vitamin D also helps lower the risk of osteoporosis, which has an increased diagnostic rate in people with MS. High levels of Vitamin D3 are shown to offer no significant side effects, while the benefits are simply remarkable.

Vitamin B1

Part of my daily regimen is to take fifty milligrams of Vitamin B1 every day, which is 3,333 percent of the recommended daily value. It has long been believed that a B1 deficiency can lead to nerve damage. Studies show that in addition to providing energy, B1 also helps balance the mood and improve heart health.

MS can actually contribute to Vitamin B1 deficiency, which can lead to damage of the myelin sheath around the nerves. Taking these supplements in large doses can help ensure your body is metabolizing enough of the vitamin, which helps to reduce nerve damage and providing relief of symptoms.

Vitamin B6

Vitamin B6 deficiency is another common deficiency in people with MS. It can present with symptoms ranging from muscle weakness to dermatitis and neuropathy. Vitamin B6 also plays a large role in your body's ability to process and absorb other vitamins and nutrients, making it essential to your overall health.

I take fifty milligrams of vitamin B6 daily, which is 2,500 percent of the recommended daily value. Studies show that a B6 deficiency can contribute to increased MS symptoms. Taking these supplements in high doses can actually help boost the nervous and immune systems, as well as aid in the production of healthy red blood cells. Taking vitamin B6 can also greatly increase energy.

Vitamin B12

My daily regimen also includes five milligrams of vitamin B12 each day. This is 83,330 percent of the recommended daily value, but studies show that this dosage offers incredible benefit without the risk of side effects. Vitamin B12 is shown to help protect the myelin sheath around the nerves, which is damaged by MS, leading to relapses and symptoms.

I first learned about vitamin B12 fairly early in my research and learned that it was supposed to be excellent for your central nervous system. At the time, I had just started a flare of my optic neuritis, which typically lasted for a couple months at a time. I started taking vitamin B12 early into the flare, and it ended up lasting only a couple weeks. I knew almost instantly that the B12 was having a positive effect on my MS.

Taking B12 can help prevent nerve damage and improve cellular longevity. A deficiency in vitamin B12 can cause vision problems, dizziness, muscle weakness, and many other symptoms. These symptoms are extremely common in people with MS, and because our bodies often do not metabolize enough of this nutrient from food, high supplement levels can offer great benefit while preventing a deficiency.

Omega 3

Omega 3 fatty acids are popular for helping to prevent a wide range of health conditions as new studies continue to prove their wide reaching health benefits. Studies have shown that the brain-boosting effects of these supplements offer great benefit for people with MS.

Patients taking Omega 3 supplements have shown fewer relapses and exacerbations of their MS, as well as a slowed progression of disability. In addition to helping behavioral and cognitive function, Omega 3 fatty acids are also shown to help reduce depression and help protect against myriad health problems and conditions.

DHA

DHA is an Omega 3 fatty acid. I take 500 milligrams daily in liquid form. It is shown to help lower the incidence rate of depression and help protect the myelin sheath. But more importantly, regular use of DHA supplements is shown to help decrease relapse frequency and improve symptoms for patients with MS. I know this has been the case for me, though I believe that a great deal of my progress lies in the combination of all of my diet, lifestyle, and vitamin and supplement changes working together. I do believe that DHA is an essential part of this.

EPA

I take 400 milligrams of EPA, another Omega 3, in liquid form every day. EPS is shown to help play a role in many cellular processes and plays a crucial part in the function and maintenance of the nervous system. When combined with DHA, they offer complementary benefits, each helping the other to be more effective in protecting the body and helping to boost the brain and nervous system.

Calcium

Calcium, a mineral essential to bone health, has also shown to benefit people with MS. Calcium helps boost the body's ability to transmit nerve impulses. Calcium also works with magnesium to help properly send nerve signals throughout the body. As part of my daily regimen, I take 1,000 milligrams of calcium, in addition to the 100 percent of the recommended daily value included in my multivitamin.

Magnesium

As mentioned, magnesium can help regulate electrical or nerve impulses throughout the body. Many patients with MS present a deficiency in magnesium, which can create an exacerbation of MS symptoms. Magnesium is shown to help reduce the relapse rate for MS patients and lower the severity of symptoms. I take 500 milligrams of magnesium daily in supplement form, which is 125 percent of the daily value.

Vitamin C

Every day, I take 5,000 milligrams of vitamin C, which is 8,335 percent of the daily recommended value. Numerous studies show that vitamin C supplements offer many benefits, including working as an antiviral and antioxidant. Most importantly for MS patients, however, vitamin C helps prevent edema, which is associated with the destruction of the myelin sheath that surrounds the nerves. People with MS are also at a higher risk of developing urinary tract infections, a risk that can be at least in part lowered by taking a vitamin C supplement regularly.

Turmeric

I mentioned turmeric in the last chapter so I won't go into too much additional detail here, but I do consider it part of my vitamin supplementation. I eat approximately one teaspoon of ground turmeric on most dinnertime meals, and the benefits have been apparent to me. One thing I would like to add about the supplement is that taking it has done wonders for my energy. Every time I eat turmeric, I get a burst of internal energy. I am not sure whether the source is mental or physical, but I find it incredibly beneficial. Rather than the feeling of a racing heart that you get with caffeine, it just leaves me feeling healthier, so I intend to keep using it on a daily basis.

Remedies and Treatments I Am Not Taking

Of course, there a number of things believed to help MS, including those that I do not choose for myself. What follows are some vitamins and supplements that are not a specific part of my daily regimen. Whether they are part of my multivitamin or simply something I have not chosen to add to my diet, it is still important to offer information about their benefits so you can make a choice for yourself based on the information available. What's best for one patient may not be exactly the same for another. Having all of the information is the best way to find what is right for you.

Choline

Choline is considered to be a part of the B vitamin family. It is shown to be very important to the central nervous system, and many people with neurological disorders are shown to have a deficiency of the vitamin. Studies show that choline, which is also found in lecithin supplements, can be instrumental in helping to protect the myelin sheath and central nervous system from damage.

Vitamins A & E

Vitamins A and E are both very important antioxidants. Free radicals, which are given off as oxygenated cells, can destroy healthy tissue within the body. These two vitamins are touted for their ability to destroy free radicals, helping to prevent or lessen damage to the nervous system.

Vitamin E also helps create proper blood circulation and prevents damage to the lining of the cells.

Ginkgo Biloba

Ginkgo Biloba is an herb that has been in use as a supplement in Eastern medicine for thousands of years. It is shown to help improve cognitive function in people with dementia, and there has been limited testing that proves it can help improve memory and concentration for people with MS. Ginkgo is also a strong antioxidant and is shown to help decrease the activity of certain immune cells that attack the myelin sheath in people with MS.

Cranberry

Cranberry is well known for its ability to help prevent and treat urinary tract infections by helping to keep certain bacteria from sticking to cells that line the urinary tract. Because urinary tract infections are so common in patients with MS and because they can have serious consequences for these patients, many doctors recommend the use of cranberry supplements to help prevent them.

Valerian

This herbal supplement is made from the root of the valerian flower. Hallmarked by a somewhat unpleasant odor, Valerian is commonly used to help people fall asleep without the need for over-the-counter or prescription drugs. Studies show that valerian can decrease the amount of time required to fall asleep without any residual effects the following morning. Since sleep deprivation can contribute to fatigue and other MS-related symptoms, Valerian is a commonly chosen supplement for those with problems sleeping.

What about Chemicals?

Just as supplements can help add to the health benefits of your diet and exercise, it is important to take the time to look at how chemicals can have an adverse effect. One thing that I learned early on in my research, which I feel everyone should be aware of, is the need to use natural and chemical-free products whenever possible. It's a fact that our skin absorbs a majority of anything we put on it, whether it's soap, shampoo, hairspray, body lotion, deodorant, perfume, or any other product that touches the skin. Most of the products on the market are laden with some of the very same chemicals you would find in common household cleaning agents. Upon learning this, I knew that it was time to make a change. If something isn't safe for consumption, it isn't safe to put on your skin either.

The chemicals that I make certain to avoid are:

Parabens

Parabens are chemicals commonly found in cosmetics, soaps, and other products. There are many reasons that these should be avoided and the general consensus is that they offer zero benefit to the body. They do, on the other hand, mimic estrogen, which can play a role in the development of breast cancer. Many healthier products on the market are now being labeled as paraben free.

Lauryl Sulfate/Sulfates

Lauryl sulfate is commonly used in many soaps, toothpaste, shampoo, and other products that we expect to *lather or foam up*. The chemical is a very cheap and effective foaming agent. Lauryl sulfate and other sulfates are actually skin irritants and serve to dry out the skin, which can actually cause damage over time. There is even talk within the medical community about a possible link with cancer, though studies are still being conducted to validate or debunk the claim. Many natural products on the market are now being labeled as sulfate or sulfite free.

Aluminum

Believe it or not, aluminum is a common ingredient in many deodorants. This ingredient should absolutely never be applied to the body. It has been linked to breast cancer and Alzheimer's, as well as a number of other brain and respiratory disorders. You can find all natural or organic deodorants that are aluminum free.

Mercury

From the time we are small, we are taught that this element is very dangerous. In fact, we are even being told now to be very careful with the new energy-saver light-bulbs, which contain only a minute trace of the chemical. Yet many of us were given dental fillings as children that were laden with the element. Mercury has the potential to do great harm to the body, especially for people with MS. It has been shown to damage the blood-brain barrier and has even been identified as a possible cause of the disease. Because of this, I had my dentist remove all of my amalgam (mercury) fillings and replace them with a new composite material.

The Bottom Line

The vitamins, minerals, and herbs outlined in this chapter are shown to offer small to great benefit for people with MS. As previously stated, it is important for you to find the supplements and dosages that work best for you. Consulting a naturopath can be very beneficial. You may even find that your doctor is willing to work with you to help find a supplement regimen that can help boost the efficacy of your drug therapy. Proper testing for vitamin levels should be done on a fairly regular basis, especially when taking high levels of vitamins. Identifying any deficiencies can help you know what supplements may be best for you. When you find the right vitamins and supplements for your body, you will almost certainly notice a drastic decrease in the symptoms and severity of your MS. Finding the right supplements was a process for me, but it was one that led me to a life, free of symptoms.

With regard to the dangerous chemicals found in our everyday cosmetic products, the truth of the matter is that most of the products you buy for cleaning, beautifying, or deodorizing your body are packed with chemicals and irritants. These ingredients can give texture, create foam, enhance fragrance, or simply act as inexpensive fillers, but while they can help keep a product's price point low, they may do so at the expense of your health. Make sure to read the labels and look for products that are labeled as organic or chemical free.

CHAPTER 7

Exercise and Staying Active

Another absolutely crucial element of MS treatment is staying active as often as possible. While rest is crucial during a relapse, particularly one with severe symptoms, when the body is healthy it is important that you do everything that you can to help keep it that way. Keeping the muscles active is important and keeping the blood flowing can help protect all body systems. When your body is in great shape, you will find that it is much easier for you to fight off the disease.

It is again important to point out that I am not a doctor, fitness professional, or physical therapist. I am just an MS patient, much like you. My exercise regimen was developed after a period of experimentation and learning what my body could and could not tolerate. What is best for me may not be what is best for you, but finding the exercise regimen that is right for your body and your disease is absolutely imperative.

You have likely heard the old saying No pain, no gain. While this is true for body builders and the like, don't use it as your motto when trying to develop an exercise regimen for MS. Pushing the body to develop stronger cardio muscles and stronger muscles in general is great, but you don't want to work out to the point of overheating or to the point of actual pain. Don't overstress your mind or your body with your workouts. If you don't work out often, slowly build your way up to a routine rather than starting with an hour of exercise every day.

What Works for Me

While we are all different, it may be helpful for you to know what I find to be the best exercise regimen for me and my MS. I typically go to the gym five days per week. This gives my body plenty of exercise without being too taxing and leaving me susceptible to relapses or exacerbations from stress and physical exhaustion.

During my visit to the gym, I try to do at least twenty minutes of stretching and warming up, thirty minutes of cardio exercise, and forty minutes of weight training. Light cardio can be a great way to warm up the body, and it helps to get the blood pumping and flowing to all your muscles. Doing cardio before your strength training helps to ensure that your blood is pumping at maximum efficiency, which greatly reduces the chances for injury and muscle strain during the weight lifting part of your regimen.

It is important to take caution not to overheat during your cardio exercise, as many MS symptoms can be exacerbated by heat. My optic neuritis can flare up whenever my body temperature rises significantly, so I know that I have to be careful not to get overheated. Learning to recognize symptoms of becoming overheated is important, and for many, it may mean finding a different way to do cardiovascular exercises outside of a hot gym.

Swimming Makes for Great Cardio

Ensuring that I do not get overheated during my cardio workouts is often simplified by the fact that I like to do my cardio in the swimming pool at the gym. The water naturally keeps my body temperature down and prevents overheating. This means that I can work out longer and harder than I would be able to do using standard cardio equipment. There are also a number of other benefits to exercising while swimming, and they are certainly worth pointing out here.

For starters, the buoyancy of water helps promote muscle relaxation. This alone can be appealing, but it also means that you have greater range of motion while in the water, offering you a more effective workout. The viscosity of the water also helps to provide resistance to all of your movements, which can help you build strength.

The resistance that water exercise provides causes you to move more slowly, which also enables you to work on both balance and coordination while swimming. The pressure of water is also greater than the air around you, providing the body with extra support. This can help make you much more flexible than you would be if you were doing the same exercises outside of the pool.

Swimming is also a form of no-impact exercise, which means it is much better for the joints than exercises such as running. While running is considered a great form of cardio, it is not recommended for those who are sensitive to heat, have muscle disabilities, or who have damage to the joints in the knees or ankles. Swimming, on the other hand, provides no impact to the joints. When combined, all these qualities offer a greater cardio workout that effectively builds endurance. Swimming is an excellent form of exercise that can boost strength, cardio health, flexibility, balance, and overall well-being.

Of course, it is also important to mention what many consider to be the biggest benefit of exercising in a swimming pool. It's fun! There are tons of exercises you can do and even just swimming regularly can provide the body with a great workout. Jumping in with kids or grandkids or taking a class can enhance the social aspect of exercise and help make it even more enjoyable.

Swimming has been exceptionally helpful for me. Spending twenty or thirty minutes in the water leaves me feeling refreshed and amazing. I feel more centered and uplifted. I know that swimming isn't always easy for those with MS, but I also know that it can have remarkable benefits on your health. When I first started, it was very difficult for me to swim for long periods of time, and I was lucky to do a few laps. Today, I can swim for over an hour without breaking for rest. With time and consistent practice, it becomes much easier and more beneficial.

Safety and Health Tips

Exercising when you have MS can be different than it is for other people. While most people can simply walk into a gym and start working out at maximum strength, many people with MS need to take precautions. What follows are a few safety tips I have picked up along the way. Some are common sense and some hold true for all people, while others are MS specific and learned only through experience. Hopefully these tips will lead you to a safer workout.

- A warm-up and cool-down period is important. This gets the muscles ready for exercise and helps release stress built up after strength training. Splitting your cardio time into half before the workout and half after can be a great strategy. It can also help keep your metabolism burning strong all day long. Be sure to incorporate stretching into your warm-up and cool-down periods.
- Always ensure that you are in a completely safe environment. Ensure that there are no tripping hazards in your workout area, avoid floors that may be slippery,

and always have a spotter if you are working with free weights.

- If you have any problems balancing at all, ensure that you are working out in an area with a rail or bar that you can use for support.

- Remember that estimated workout times and goals are not crucial. While you certainly want to exercise a certain amount of time with each workout, your health and safety come first. If the workout becomes painful or you start to feel ill, stop what you are doing immediately and rest. You can always exercise another day; pushing your body too hard can be counterproductive.

- Avoid working out during the hottest times of day, especially if you are heat sensitive. Exercise in the morning or evening instead.

- If you notice that you are starting to overheat or that you are having new symptoms, stop exercising immediately and allow the body to cool down.

- ALWAYS bring a bottle of water with you to the gym or wherever you work out. Drink plenty of cool fluids throughout your workout and the entire day to help prevent overheating and to keep you hydrated. Water is a key ingredient to protecting and healing the body.

Exercise Doesn't Have to Be Boring

One thing that keeps many people with MS from developing the exercise habits that they need is the feeling or boredom or work that many associate with working out.

While exercise can be hard work, that doesn't mean it can't also be enjoyable. If you find you cannot stick to a traditional cardio and strength-training regimen, why not consider other options? Giving up on the notion of exercise entirely can be devastating to your health and your MS. Finding a fun alternative to those trips to the gym can be a much better option.

One great choice can be to find a workout buddy. It can be someone you know who shares your diagnosis, a family member, or a friend. Find someone else who wants to get into better shape and go to the gym together. Conversation can make any workout less stressful. If that isn't right for you, you can also consider taking a class. Most gyms offer a variety of classes, including water aerobics. You will also find that classes such as tai chi and yoga can offer a good workout that also improves balance, coordination, and strength without overheating or overtiring the body.

Sleep Is Important, Too

Believe it or not, a healthy sleep regimen is as essential to your workouts and your health as the exercises themselves. Sleep is when our bodies recuperate from not only mental stress but physical stress as well. Exercise puts strain on your muscles, and it is when you are sleeping that your body takes the time to heal, rest, and recover. I try for a minimum of seven hours of sleep a night. I go to bed early each night and get up at 4:30 A.M. during the week so that I can go to the gym before work. On the weekends I try to sleep a little longer, which helps me get the extra rest I need after a busy week.

The Bottom Line

Exercise is an imperative for the MS patient. It has led to better health for me and has contributed immeasurably to a life that is free of MS symptoms. When combined with other lifestyle and diet changes, it can help to do the same for you. The benefits of exercise are big for everyone, but when you have a disease that can be disabling, they become even more important. I would like to close this chapter with some research and facts regarding the link between MS and exercise.

In 2010, Ohio State University conducted studies examining the difference between MS patients who were considered to be highly physically fit and patients who exhibited the same levels of the disease and who fit into the same demographics, but were less physically fit. The study showed that those who were physically fit performed significantly better on cognitive function tests. They also showed considerably less damage and deterioration in areas of the brain affected by MS, showing far less atrophy and presented with a higher volume of gray matter. The conclusion of the study was that physical fitness helps to protect gray matter and the areas of the brain that are most affected by MS, proving that the link between MS and fitness is indeed a very strong one.

The very first study to conclusively prove the link between exercise and an improvement for patients with MS was conducted in 1996 by researchers at the University of Utah. That study clearly showed that patients who participated in aerobic exercises showed better cardiovascular fitness, greater strength, a lower instance of both fatigue and depression, higher bladder and bowel function, and a more positive and social attitude. Since that study, these benefits have been confirmed numerous times.

Exercising can certainly help reduce the frequency and severity of relapses and exacerbations, but it can also do much more. In addition to helping improve mental health and mood, exercise can prevent coronary heart disease, muscle weakness, and decreased bone density, all of which are more common in people with MS. While patients with severe or progressed cases may need to work with a physical therapist to find a workout that is healthy and safe, evidence of the benefits of exercise is too strong to be ignored.

Caring for your body and eliminating symptoms of your MS takes a great deal of effort on your part, and exercise is an instrumental part of this. You don't have to let MS control your life. Finding a workout that you enjoy and that really exercises your muscles can offer significant benefit. I know that my exercise habits are a major part of why I am able to live a life free of MS symptoms and why my disease has actually regressed instead of progressing. By finding a program that works for you, a life without symptoms or with significantly reduced symptoms of MS is a possibility for you, too.

CHAPTER 8

Staying on Track

If there is one thing I know about making radical changes to your lifestyle, it is that it is not easy. Reading about all the things that are possible if you make these changes can be a great motivator. You will seriously start thinking about how much different your life can be, but you need to know that it is still going to be hard work. I'm not sure that anyone thinks about making all of these changes and then wakes up every day excited to exercise, cut out foods that he or she loves, and take a ton of vitamins and supplements. To be honest, some days it really does feel like forcing yourself to do it. Understand that this will happen but that the end result is worth the effort.

Motivation is not about waking up every day and wanting to make all of the right choices. If it was, few people could truly call themselves motivated. Instead, motivation is about waking up every day and doing them anyway.

While exercising, eating all of the right foods, skipping the wrong foods, and taking vitamins every day is crucial, it is not easy to do every day without fail. You have to find a routine that works for you, and more importantly, you have to stick to it. Exercising sporadically, occasionally eating right, or taking your supplements only when you remember is not going to help your body repair itself and fight off the symptoms of MS. You need a routine that you can stick to without fail and that your body can adjust to. Otherwise, you are just creating confusion for your mind and body.

Resolving to make changes in your life is easy but finding the internal resolve to make them stick is much harder. The good news is that you can make these things a part of your daily life. After a few weeks of a new routine, it is much easier to get up and do the same things every day. Your body will create a habit and will adjust to these changes, but you have to do them with consistency to ensure this happens.

After a couple of weeks on an MS friendly diet you will start feeling more energetic and healthier. This can make it much easier to stick to this aspect of your new routine. Making a switch back to unhealthy foods or to those that trigger symptoms will leave you feeling ill, lethargic, or just plain awful. You will quickly discover that a proper diet is the best way to live a healthy, symptom-free life. You can easily find alternatives for your favorite foods that don't include trigger ingredients but still offer the flavor that you have come to enjoy.

Exercise is another hard part of your lifestyle to change. For many people, the notion of exercising can fill them with dread, and it is perhaps the easiest part of the routine to skip. It is impossible to overstress the importance of exercise. You absolutely have to find a way to get yourself moving every day.

The good news when looking to stay motivated with a new exercise regimen is that after even a few minutes of cardio you have more energy than when you began, and your body and mind will feel considerably better. Exercise is a natural stress buster, which can leave you feeling healthier and refreshed even after a few minutes.

Taking vitamins and supplements can also be a hard change to implement. Even though taking all your supplements is an easy task, it can also be easy to simply forget. Unfortunately, to build a consistent level of vitamins and minerals in the blood, you have to remember to take them every day and throughout the day, not all at once.

Setting an alarm for the same times every day and taking your supplements as soon as the alarm goes off can help make this part of your routine. With time, this will become part of your muscle memory, and you will be able to remember to take your supplements each day without the need for an alarm. Setting a time right before or after a meal can make it easier for you to remember. I have made it easy for myself and take my vitamins and supplements with breakfast, lunch, and dinner.

Staying Motivated

While telling you how to motivate yourself is simple, I know that actually finding the motivation can be hard. I have made all of these changes myself, and I can assure you that I didn't just wake up every day thinking "I can't wait to work out and eat only specific foods." While I love my routine now and stick to it daily, it wasn't always so simple. I know what goes through your mind on the mornings that you just feel exhausted. The good news is that my experience can help you avoid some of the pitfalls that I experienced.

By far, one of the best pieces of advice that I can offer is not to set your goals too high right off the bat. If you create an initial goal of working out an hour a day and losing a large amount of weight, you are setting yourself up for disappointment. These are certainly excellent long-term goals, but you will find it is much easier to achieve success by setting smaller and more easily accomplished goals. Create goals that you can reach in a relatively short period of time, and the feeling of success can help you stay motivated.

Aim for fifteen to twenty minutes of exercise daily to start, and work hard to achieve it. When that goal is achieved and that amount of exercise has become easily tolerated for you, set your goal a little higher. You don't have to reach peak health and fitness tomorrow for your regimen to be effective. Don't push yourself to do too much too soon, start slow. Otherwise it is going to be all but impossible for you to want to or be able to stick to an exercise or diet regimen.

Another great tip is to learn to substitute. If you simply cut all your favorite foods out of your diet, you are not going to enjoy it or find yourself nearly as driven to stick to it. Can't eat gluten but love pasta? Try some of the great gluten-free pasta noodles out there, which are brown rice based. They taste remarkably similar to your old pasta and allow you to keep enjoying those favorite foods.

Another very important tip is to design a schedule that accommodates your changing goals. If you already lead a very busy life and suddenly find yourself trying to fit an hour of exercise into the exact same schedule, you are going to find yourself on the road to burn out. Look for little things that you can shorten or cut out of your day. Consider getting up a little bit earlier or even consider working out on your lunch break or during other times that you are free. Ensure that your schedule is designed for your new lifestyle so that doing these new things doesn't take away from time you already have scheduled for other tasks.

Many people find that writing down their goals can be helpful. Write down the changes you want to make and write down what you want to accomplish. Write down what types of bodily changes you hope to see from a new diet and exercise plan, what types of MS symptom reductions you can achieve with a more balanced lifestyle, and even the emotional effects of a healthier regimen. Writing down what you have to look forward to can help make it more tangible. Read what you have written every day to help keep you motivated. This will help you remember what you can accomplish by sticking to this regimen, even when the going gets tough.

The biggest thing to remember when it comes to your new goals is that you have to stick with them even after the honeymoon period is over. When you first set goals for a new diet, exercise, and supplement regimen, you have a clear notion of a healthier life that is free of MS symptoms. For the first few days, you are likely to experience a feeling that is almost a high, as you get ready to exercise and eat healthy foods that will benefit your body. This is great, but you need to understand that not every day will feel like this.

The feeling of starting a new routine or regimen is almost like the feeling you get when falling in love. It is all very thrilling at first but eventually you learn that to keep it going, you have to put in some hard work. The same is true for changing your lifestyle. If you accept this and find the willingness to see your regimen through even the toughest times, you are much more likely to see long-term success.

The Bottom Line

Sticking with your new regimen is going to be hard. No matter how fun your workout routine and no matter how delicious your new diet may be there will be days when you simply don't wake up and think about how much you can't wait to work out. The key is to do it anyway. You need to know that there will be days where exercise and healthy foods will be the last thing you want, so you need to prepare for this. You don't want to wake up like unenthusiastic for your new regimen and have no idea how to handle it.

I have been aggressively following my regimen for many years now. It isn't always fun and exciting, but it is always worthwhile. Over the years my symptoms and side effects have lessened considerably and now, I don't have them at all.

In many ways I feel as though I have overcome MS by taking my medication and vitamins, sticking to my diet, exercising, and living the healthiest life I can possibly live. But I also know that all of this can be undone if I stop adhering to my regimen. At the end of the day, there is still no real cure for MS. My lifestyle keeps the disease at bay and helps me live a symptom-free life. I know that if I give up my routine, it can show up full force tomorrow. When all else fails and when I have days where I simply don't feel like working out, it is this knowledge that helps keep me motivated and on my regimen. A life free of symptoms and relapses is always going to be worth an hour spent exercising or a diet that eliminates unhealthy ingredients.

CHAPTER 9

Find a Support System

Finding a good support system is incredibly important for anyone, especially for people diagnosed with MS. As a patient myself, I know how hard it can be to deal with this illness, especially in the beginning when you have so many worries and questions. Dealing with the diagnosis of MS can be very hard, particularly if you are trying to do it alone.

When I was first diagnosed, I felt as though nobody in my life could understand how it felt to have this disease. In many ways I still feel this way. I have learned I do not want them to understand how I feel or how I felt at my worst. In order to know what it really feels like to have this disease, you have to experience it, and that is something I don't wish on anyone.

You will learn a lot about the disease in the time after you are first diagnosed with MS. In many ways, you will mature in your expectations of the people around you. While a support system within the MS community is immeasurably helpful, you will find that the support of family and friends can be exceptionally helpful. Even if they don't know what it is like to live with this disease, it is important to have the support of loved ones.

The people closest to me may not know what living with MS is like, but they are always available for me to talk to. My wife, my parents, my sister, and my mother-in-law are there to listen to me discuss my life and my feelings. Their support is an instrumental part of my life. I found that in the beginning I didn't want to talk about the disease because I felt that doing so would mean admitting that I had MS. Eventually, I had to come to terms with the diagnosis and having people there to support me made it much easier.

Today, I understand my MS. I understand what the disease is and how it affects me and other people who have been diagnosed. I am no longer afraid or ashamed to have the disease, and I am not ashamed for other people to know that I have Multiple Sclerosis. Instead, I find that I am incredibly proud of all that I have achieved and how hard I have fought to get where I am today. I am also happy to share my story so that I can help others experience the same successes, without the struggles I experienced along the way.

It is crucial that you have people in your life that you can talk to. You need to be able to share your stories, your pain, and your emotions. You need to be able to share your hopes and your triumphs. Allow your loved ones to be part of your support system and allow them to help you manage the disease.

It may not be easy to open up to others and there will certainly be times that you feel like no one really understands, but realize that sometimes simply caring for you is enough. Even when your loved ones don't understand what it is like to not have enough energy to simply make breakfast in the morning, they can support you when you are feeling that way. Having a support system is crucial. You will find that it can offer you what you need to keep going whenever times are tough and also provide someone with whom to share your triumphs.

Learning how to be completely open about the disease can be difficult. You may also find that it can be hard knowing exactly in whom you should confide. Understand that needing a shoulder to lean on now and then is not a weakness; it is a part of the human experience. We all need the ability to talk, to express, and to have someone with whom to share our burdens. The bottom line is that the love and support from people closest to you can make the fight easier.

Extend Your Network

The support of family members and friends can certainly be of immeasurable help, but connecting with other people who share your diagnosis also can be very important.

When I first began accepting my diagnosis, I started visiting online MS forums. I learned that talking with other people who shared the diagnosis was a great way to share stories, find people who understand what life with MS is like on a daily basis, and vent when things start to feel hopeless.

There are people all over the world who are going through the same things and have gotten through the toughest times and come out on the other side happier, healthier, and more experienced. Connecting with others who share your diagnosis and who have a positive attitude can be an important part of your own growth and progress. It is something that I recommend for everyone.

The Bottom Line

While it may be possible to go through this alone, I do not recommend it. Opening yourself up to loved ones makes it easier for them to understand you and offer the support you need. If you find that you don't want advice, you can simply tell them so. Allowing loved ones to take this journey with you is important. They may not understand everything that you go through but simply having someone to walk alongside with and hold your hand when you need it, can make a world of difference. Connect with loved ones, connect with strangers, and connect with whomever you choose, but don't go through this alone.

I also recommend sharing this book with your loved ones. Ask them to read this book so they can gain a deep understanding for the disease and what you may be going through. Having them understand MS and the symptoms and emotions that come along with it is very important and can make their level of support much stronger.

CHAPTER 10

Change Your Mindset Starting Now

Living with MS is not easy. For some people, living with this disease means being in pain more often than not or being so tired that you cannot do the things you need to do, let alone the things that you want to do. For some people, vision problems can be severe and others find themselves in need of a cane or a wheelchair to get around. For others, life can feel hopeless or like too much of a struggle to keep going on.

I know how bad it can be to live with MS on the rough days, and I know how bad it can hurt both physically and emotionally. But I also know that we have within ourselves the ability to fight this disease. If you are willing to let MS get the best of you, it will. But if you commit yourself to beating it and to making it something that you can live with, you can do that as well.

There will be days that you feel great, and you think, there's nothing to this. But there will also be days when getting the motivation to do the things you need to do will take everything you've got—I know, I've been there. I've been at complete rock bottom, and I have spent my fair share of days believing that there was nothing to get up for, that life wasn't worth continuing. I spent a lot of time in that space, but through it all, I kept fighting.

Even when things were at their toughest, I kept researching this disease, eating all the right foods, taking different vitamins and supplements to see what would work for me, and going to the gym five days a week. I pushed through even when it was the last thing I wanted to do. I know that this is the reason I am here now, in control of the disease, rather than it in control of me.

The same year I was diagnosed with MS, I also started my own business. That meant that even while I was still learning about this disease and fighting with the symptoms, I was also trying to focus on getting my own business off the ground and waiting tables at night to ensure that there was a roof over my head. But through all of this, I kept on fighting. It's what I do. I refuse to let anything get the best of me, including this disease.

Every day, I know that I only have one life to enjoy here on earth. Once my cards have been dealt, there is no trading them in. This is the hand I was given, and I choose to play it rather than fold. I do everything I can to enjoy not only a successful life, but a happy one as well. In the years since I was diagnosed, I have managed to build a successful company and marry the woman I love. My wife and I are getting ready to welcome our first baby into the world. I am successful in business and life, and I am successful with my MS. My life is more than manageable—it is happy, productive, and blessed.

I know that despite my disease, I will continue to make things happen. This is my first book, but I know that there will be more to come. I plan to start more businesses. Most importantly, I will always do my best to ensure that I live a happy and healthy life for my family and me. We can accomplish anything in this world. For those of us with MS, it means having the right motivation and determination, the right conventional and nonconventional medicine, the right vitamins and supplements, the right diet and lifestyle, and above all, the right attitude. We can do anything even while living with a disabling disease.

One thing that you must always remember is that you are not alone in this fight. There are hundreds of thousands of people all over the world fighting with you. I am fighting with you. In the moments where everything feels the toughest, I want you to dig down deep, find the strength you need to fight this disease, and create for yourself a life that is filled with health, success, happiness, and love.

I hope that you have found my story helpful. I do not offer you this story as one that you should compare to your own, but as one that can help you see a bit of me within yourself or a bit of yourself in me and my story. I hope that you can use my experience and my research to uncover a newfound light that will guide you to a better life, as you go on to live with MS.

I offer an open invitation to anyone who has read this to reach out and contact me. Whether you want to ask questions, get my opinion, give or receive advice, share experiences, or if you just need someone to provide you with a shoulder to lean on, I urge you to do so.

You can contact me anytime via my Web site at www.MSLivingSymptomFree.com

I wish you a long, healthy, and happy life.

From one MS patient to another,

Daryl

APPENDIX 1

All Natural MS-Friendly Recipes – Free of Gluten, Dairy, and Legumes

While I have spent a great deal of time explaining my diet, I also know that telling someone what kind of lifestyle I maintain, without providing an example of how someone else can maintain and achieve it, is not always helpful. In this section, you will find more than twenty-five of my favorite all natural MS-friendly recipes. Each recipe in this section is free of gluten, dairy, and legumes but offers plenty of flavor. I enjoy these meals on a regular basis and am confident that you will enjoy them as well. Even if these recipes don't seem right for you, they can help offer some suggestions for what to look for in an all-natural MS-friendly diet.

SOUPS

Turkey Rice Soup

Ingredients:

- Leftover turkey parts with meat (wings, drumsticks, legs)
- Peppercorns
- 4 celery stalks, sliced
- Bay leaves
- Half an onion, quartered
- 4 carrots, sliced
- Celery, chopped
- Onions, chopped
- Thyme (fresh or dry)
- Gluten-free chicken bouillon (or no bouillon and substitute water with chicken or vegetable stock)
- 2 cups cooked brown rice

Directions:

1. Place all leftover turkey and turkey bones in pot, and cover with water. Add bay leaves and peppercorns to pot. Cover and cook on medium heat for 90 minutes or until meat begins to fall off bone.
2. Remove turkey meat. Cool meat then pick off bones and set aside.

3. Add carrots, celery, and onion. Add thyme, salt, pepper, and bouillon. Cook until veggies are soft.
4. Return turkey meat to pot and cook an additional 20 minutes.
5. Put rice in bowl and ladle turkey soup on top. Serve and enjoy.

Hearty Hot or Cold Roasted Tomato Soup

Ingredients:

- 2 pounds Roma (plum) tomatoes, quartered
- 3 tablespoons olive oil
- 4 cloves garlic
- 1 quart chicken stock
- ¼ cup chopped fresh basil
- ½ T balsamic vinegar
- Salt to taste
- Ground black pepper to taste

Directions:

1. Place the tomato halves, cut side up, on a baking tray with the garlic cloves. Drizzle with the oil, and sprinkle with salt and pepper. Roast at 375 degrees F (195 degrees C) for 1 hour.
2. Snip the ends off the garlic cloves, and squeeze the insides into the bowl of a food processor, along with the entire contents of the baking tray. Add stock, basil, and vinegar; blend until smooth. Season to taste.
3. Serve either hot or cold.

This recipe is courtesy of Rosa on allrecipes.com

Grandma's Chicken and Vegetable Soup

Ingredients:

- 1 large whole chicken
- 2 bay leaves
- Peppercorns
- 1 cup chopped onion
- ½ cup chopped celery
- ½ cup chopped carrot
- 1 T thyme
- Salt and pepper to taste
- 1 gluten-free chicken bouillon (or no bouillon and substitute water with chicken or vegetable stock)

Directions:

1. Place the chicken in a large boiling pot of water with celery, onions, carrots, bay leaf, and peppercorns; cover with water. Cover pot with lid and boil on medium heat until chicken is cooked through.
2. Remove chicken and set aside to cool. Add thyme, salt, pepper, and gluten-free chicken bouillon.
3. After chicken has cooled, remove meat from the bone. Put all chicken pieces in the pot and simmer for an additional 20 minutes. Serve as is or over rice and enjoy.

Simple Carrot Ginger Soup

Original Recipe Yield 6 Servings

Ingredients:

- 3 T olive oil
- 1 yellow or white onion, chopped
- ¼ cup peeled and finely chopped ginger root
- 3 cloves garlic, minced
- 6 cups vegetable or chicken stock
- 1 ½ pounds carrots, peeled and cut into 1/2 inch chunks
- 1 t turmeric (optional)
- Salt and ground pepper
- Optional garnishes: chives or parsley

Directions:

1. Sauté onion, ginger, and garlic in olive oil for 5-10 minutes.
2. Add the stock and carrots, and bring to boil. Reduce heat and simmer uncovered over medium heat until the carrots are very tender, about 30 minutes.
3. Puree the soup with an immersion blender or in batches in a blender or food processor.
4. Season with turmeric, and salt and pepper to taste. Serve and enjoy.

Salads

Mediterranean Salad

Original Recipe Yield 4 Servings

Ingredients:

- 3 tablespoons extra virgin olive oil, divided
- ¼ t sea salt
- 6 cups organic arugula (about 4 ounces)
- 1 cup thinly sliced green onions
- ½ cup tomatoes, chopped
- ¼ cup thinly sliced basil leaves
- 1 ½ T balsamic vinegar

Directions:

1. Combine arugula, green onions, basil, vinegar, toma-toes, and 3 tablespoons olive oil in large bowl and toss. Season with salt and pepper.
2. Divide greens among plates.

Greek Salad

Original Recipe Yield 4 Servings

Ingredients:

- 1 cup tomato, diced
- 2 T red wine vinegar
- 2 T extra virgin olive oil
- ½ seedless cucumber, halved lengthwise, cored, and diced (1 cup)
- ½ cup pitted kalamata olives, slivered
- ¼ cup thinly sliced red onion
- 2 T fresh lemon juice
- 2 T chopped flat-leaf parsley
- 1 T finely chopped oregano
- 2 to 3 cups coarsely chopped romaine
- 4 to 8 pepperoncini

Directions:

1. Toss together tomato, parsley, vinegar, 1 tablespoon oil, salt, and pepper. Set aside and marinate in refrigerator for 15 minutes.
2. Toss together remaining tablespoon oil, cucumber, olives, onion, lemon juice, and oregano in a large bowl.
3. Blend all ingredients together and divide mixture among plates on top of romaine lettuce.
4. Add 1 or 2 pepperoncini to each plate.

Apple Pecan Chicken Spinach Salad

Original Recipe Yield 4 Servings

Ingredients:

- 8 cups spinach
- 1 ½ cup cooked, shredded rotisserie chicken breast
- ¼ cup chopped pecans, toasted
- Red onion, sliced very thin
- Tomatoes
- 4 medium apples, chopped

Apple White Balsamic Vinaigrette

- 2 T apple juice concentrate
- 1 T apple cider vinegar
- 1 T white balsamic vinegar
- 1 t Dijon mustard
- ¼ t garlic powder
- ¼ 3cup olive oil

Directions:

1. Toss spinach, chicken, onion, tomato, pecans, and apple together in a large salad bowl.
2. Whisk together remaining ingredients and pour over salad. Serve immediately and enjoy.

Spinach and Avocado Salad with Balsamic Vinaigrette

Original Recipe Yield 3 Servings

Ingredients:

- 1 bag fresh spinach, about 10 to 12 ounces
- ½ cup tomatoes, chopped
- 1 avocado, sliced
- ½ cup balsamic vinegar
- ½ tsp. sea salt
- ½ t oregano
- ¼ cup olive oil

Directions:

1. Wash spinach and let dry. Whisk together vinegar, oil, sea salt, and oregano. Refrigerate spinach and dressing separately until serving time.
2. Add chopped tomatoes and avocado. Pour dressing over salad just before serving and toss.

Sides and Appetizers

Guacamole

Original Recipe Yield 3 Servings

Ingredients:

- 2 ripe Hass avocados
- 1 lime, juiced
- ½ small onion, chopped
- 1 garlic clove, minced
- 1 jalapeño, chopped
- 1 handful fresh cilantro leaves, roughly chopped
- Sea salt and freshly ground black pepper
- Drizzle of olive oil

Directions:

1. Halve and pit the avocados. With a tablespoon, scoop out flesh of the avocado and place in a mixing bowl. Mash the avocados with a fork, leaving them still a bit chunky.
2. Add the rest of the ingredients, and mix or fold everything together.
3. Place plastic wrap on top of guacamole (so it doesn't brown) and chill in refrigerator before serving.

Quick Sautéed Kale with Garlic

Original Recipe Yield 3 Servings

Ingredients:

- 1 bunch organic kale
- 4 T olive oil
- 2 garlic cloves, minced

Directions:

1. Fold each kale leaf lengthwise in half; cut stem away along crease. Tear leaves coarsely.
2. Heat oil in heavy large pot over medium heat. Add garlic; heat for about 3 minutes, careful not to burn garlic.
3. Add kale. Cook until kale wilts slightly, tossing often, every 2 to 3 minutes.
4. Season to taste with salt and pepper. Transfer to bowl.

Quinoa Side Dish

Original Recipe Yield 4 Servings

Ingredients:

- 1 T butter
- 1 cup uncooked quinoa
- 2 cups vegetable broth
- 2 t chopped garlic
- 2 T chopped fresh parsley
- ½ T chopped fresh thyme
- ¼ t salt
- 1 small onion, finely chopped
- 1 dash fresh lemon juice (optional)

Directions:

1. Melt butter in a saucepan over medium heat. Add the quinoa, and toast, stirring occasionally, until lightly browned, about 5 minutes. Stir in broth, and bring to a boil. Reduce to a simmer, cover, and cook for 15 minutes, or until quinoa is tender.
2. In a bowl, toss quinoa together with garlic, parsley, thyme, salt, and onion. Sprinkle with lemon juice, and serve.

This recipe is courtesy of Sal on allrecipes.com

Sautéed Asparagus with Garlic

Original Recipe Yield 4 Servings

Ingredients:

- ½ pound fresh asparagus, trimmed
- 2 T water
- 1 T olive oil
- 2 garlic cloves, chopped or minced
- ⅛ t salt
- 1 dash white or black pepper

Directions:

1. Place asparagus and water in pan and heat on stove for 5 minutes over medium heat.
2. Combine olive oil, garlic, salt, and pepper. Drizzle over asparagus and toss to coat.

Heat for an additional 5 minutes until desired tenderness is reached.

Baked Sweet Potatoes with Ginger and Honey

Original Recipe Yield 12 Servings (cut ingredients in half to reduce servings to 6)

Ingredients:

- 9 sweet potatoes, peeled and cubed
- ½ cup honey
- 3 T grated fresh ginger
- 2 T walnut oil
- 1 t ground cardamom
- ½ t ground black pepper

Directions:

1. Preheat oven to 400 degrees (205 degrees C).
2. In a large bowl, combine the sweet potatoes, honey, ginger, oil, cardamom, and pepper. Transfer to a large cast iron frying pan. Bake for 20 minutes.
3. Turn the mixture over to expose the pieces from the bottom of the pan. Bake for another 20 minutes, or until the sweet potatoes are tender and caramelized on the outside.

This recipe is courtesy of Christine L. on allrecipes.com

Roasted Brussels Sprouts

Original Recipe Yield 6 Servings

Ingredients:

- 1 ½ pounds Brussels sprouts, ends trimmed and yellow leaves removed
- 3 T olive oil
- 1 t kosher salt
- ½ t freshly ground black pepper

Directions:

1. Preheat oven to 400 degrees F (205 degrees C).
2. Place trimmed Brussels sprouts, olive oil, kosher salt, and pepper in a large resealable plastic bag. Seal tightly, and shake to coat. Pour onto a baking sheet, and place on center oven rack.
3. Roast in the preheated oven for 30 to 45 minutes, shaking pan every 5 to 7 minutes for even browning. Reduce heat when necessary to prevent burning. Brussels sprouts should be dark brown, almost black, when done. Adjust seasoning with kosher salt, if necessary. Serve immediately.

This recipe is courtesy of JAQATAC on allrecipes.com

Entrees – Breakfast

Avocado and Onion Egg White Omelet

Original Recipe Yield 1 Omelet

Ingredients:

- 3 large egg whites
- ½ avocado
- ½ medium white onion, sliced or diced
- 2 tablespoons olive oil
- Sea salt and pepper to taste

Directions:

1. Put 2 tablespoons olive oil and onions into pan or skillet over medium head. Cook onions for a few minutes.
2. Pour egg whites into skillet and continue cooking until egg is fully cooked.
3. Add avocado to half of egg. Flip the other half of the egg over the top to make the omelet
4. Remove from heat and enjoy!

For a spicy omelet, add ½ fresh jalapeno or ½ teaspoon red pepper flakes

Gluten-Free Pancakes

Original Recipe Yield 4 Servings

Ingredients:

- 1 egg
- ¾ cup gluten-free baking mix
- 1 ½ t baking soda
- 1 T canola oil
- 1 t gluten-free baking powder
- ¾ cup water
- ¼ cup tapioca flour (not starch)

Directions:

1. Beat egg in bowl with fork. Sift together baking soda, baking powder, baking mix, and tapioca flour. Mix all ingredients together and let stand for 5 minutes.
2. Fry on 375-degree skillet until done. Best if flipped only once.

Add chocolate chips to pancake batter for a little treat.

Gluten-Free Granola with Fruit

Original Recipe Yield 1 Serving

Ingredients:

- ½ cup gluten-free granola
- ½ cup almond, rice, or hemp milk
- ¼ cup fresh sliced strawberries
- ¼ cup fresh sliced banana

Directions:

1. Add granola and fresh fruit to breakfast bowl
2. Add almond, rice, or hemp milk.

Gluten-Free Banana Nut Oatmeal

Original Recipe Yield 1 Serving

Ingredients:

- 1 packet gluten-free oatmeal
- ¼ cup almond, rice, or hemp milk
- ½ cup fresh sliced banana
- ¼ cup walnuts

Directions:

1. Add oatmeal, almond milk, banana, and walnuts to breakfast bowl.
2. Microwave for 1–1 ½ minutes and enjoy!

Entrees – Lunch

** see salads and soups above**

Gluten-Free AB & J

Original Recipe Yield 1 Sandwich

Ingredients:

- 2 slices gluten-free bread (like Ezekiel)
- All natural fruit preserves
- All natural almond butter

Directions:

1. Toast bread slices.
2. Put almond butter on one side and fruit preserves on other. Put slices together and enjoy with your favorite gluten-free chips.

Fresh Fruit Protein Smoothie

Original Recipe Yield 4 Cups

Ingredients:

- 1 cup fresh fruit (organic blueberries, pineapple, etc…)
- 1 cup almond milk (you may also use rice or hemp milk)
- 1 scoop hemp or brown rice protein powder
- 4 ice cubes

Directions:

1. Combine milk, fresh fruit, protein powder, and ice cubes in a blender.
2. Blend until smooth.

Gluten-Free English Muffin Pizzas

Original Recipe Yield 1 Serving

Ingredients

- 1 gluten-free English muffin
- ½ cup dairy-free mozzarella cheese, shredded
- 2 T of marinara sauce
- Pepperoni or other toppings (optional)

Directions:

1. Slice English muffin. Place tomato sauce and then the mozzarella cheese on each half of the English muffin.
2. Top your pizza with a few pepperoni slices or other favorite pizza toppings.
3. Preheat oven to 350 F. Place your completed pizzas on an aluminum foil-lined baking sheet in oven or toaster oven.
4. Bake for approximately 7-10 minutes, depending on how crispy you like your pizza and until cheese is fully melted.

Entrees – Dinner

Seared Wild Salmon with Broccolini, Olives, and Garlic

Original Recipe Yield 2 Servings

Ingredients:

- 3 T extra virgin olive oil, plus additional for drizzling
- 1 bunch broccolini
- ¼ cup water
- 2 large garlic cloves, chopped
- ¼ cup halved pitted black olives
- 2 6-8 oz. wild salmon fillets with skin on (each about 1/2 to 3/4 inch thick)
- 2 T (or more) balsamic vinegar

Directions:

1. Heat 2 tablespoons oil in large skillet over medium heat. Add broccolini and stir for 1 minute. Pour 1/4 cup water, cover, and steam for 5 minutes until broccolini is crisp and tender. Add olives and garlic and stir for 1 minute. Turn off heat and set aside in bowl.
2. Heat 1 tablespoon oil in same skillet (not cleaned) over medium heat. Season salmon with salt and pepper on both sides and add fillets, skin down, and cook until skin is crisp, about 3-4 minutes. Turn salmon fillets over and cook another 2 minutes, careful not to overcook.

3. Transfer salmon fillets to plate. Return brocoolini mixture to same skillet on medium heat and add 1 tablespoon balsamic vinegar. Season to taste with salt and pepper.
4. Spoon mixture to plate with salmon. Drizzle fish lightly with oil and 1 tablespoon balsamic vinegar.
5. Serve and enjoy.

Maple Salmon

Original Recipe Yield 4 Servings

Ingredients:

- ¼ cup maple syrup
- 2 T gluten free soy sauce
- 1 clove garlic, minced
- ¼ t garlic salt
- Black pepper to taste
- 1 pound salmon

Directions

1. In a small bowl, mix the maple syrup, soy sauce, garlic, garlic salt, and pepper.
2. Place salmon in a shallow glass baking dish, and coat with the maple syrup mixture. Cover the dish, and marinate salmon in the refrigerator 30 minutes, turning once.
3. Preheat oven to 400 degrees F (200 degrees C).
4. Place the baking dish in the preheated oven, and bake salmon uncovered 20 minutes, or until easily flaked with a fork.

This recipe is courtesy of STARFLOWER on allrecipes.com

Chipotle Crusted Pork Tenderloin

Original Recipe Yield 6 Servings

Ingredients:

- 1 t onion powder
- 1 t garlic powder
- 3 T chipotle chile powder
- 1 ½ te salt
- 4 T brown sugar
- 2 (¾ pound) pork tenderloins

Directions:

1. Preheat grill for medium-high heat.
2. In a large resealable plastic bag, combine the onion powder, garlic powder, chipotle chile powder, salt, and brown sugar. Place tenderloins in bag and shake, coating meat evenly. Refrigerate for 10 to 15 minutes.
3. Lightly oil grill grate and arrange meat on grate. Cook for 20 minutes, turning meat every 5 minutes. Remove from grill, let stand for 5 to 10 minutes before slicing.

This recipe is courtesy of KRAMNODROG on allrecipes.com

Chicken Vegetable Stir-Fry

Original Recipe Yield 4 Servings

Ingredients:

- 1 pound chicken breast, cut in 1-inch cubes
- 3 T olive oil
- 1 medium onion, sliced
- 1 cup chopped asparagus
- 1 red bell pepper, sliced
- 1 cup broccoli florets
- 4 green onions, cut in ¾ inch pieces
- ½ cup water
- 2 T gluten free soy sauce
- 1 T cornstarch
- ½ t ginger minced (or ½ t ground ginger)

Directions

1. Mix water, cornstarch, soy sauce, and ginger in a small bowl and set aside.
2. Stir-fry chicken in a large skillet or wok with olive oil 3 minutes or until chicken is no longer pink.
3. Add onions, peppers, and asparagus. Stir-fry and additional 3 minutes.
4. Add broccoli, and then pour gravy mixture over chicken and vegetables and stir-fry for additional 3 minutes.
5. Stir-fry until vegetables are cooked, yet still tender crisp, serve and enjoy.

Chicken and Rice

Original Recipe Yield 6 Servings

Ingredients:

- 2 lbs. of chicken, cut into small pieces
- 4 T. extra virgin olive oil
- 1 chopped onion
- 2 garlic cloves, chopped
- Salt and pepper
- Handful fresh parsley, coarsely chopped
- 1 chopped red bell pepper
- 1 t turmeric
- 1 t paprika
- 2 ½ cups of chicken broth
- ½ cup dry white wine
- 1 ½ cups brown rice

Directions:

1. Sprinkle the chicken with salt and pepper. In a large deep pan (rice will be cooked there, too) heat the oil and sauté the chicken until golden on all sides. Remove chicken to a warm platter.
2. Add onion, garlic, and parsley to the oil, and sauté until the onion is soft and translucent. Add the turmeric, saffron, broth, wine, salt, and pepper and bring to a boil.

3. Add the rice and cook over medium high heat, uncovered, for about 20 minutes, stirring frequently until the rice is cooked.
4. Add chicken burry below rice. Cover and cook over low heat for 10 minutes. Turn the rice and the chicken over with a fork. Cover and simmer for another 10 minutes.
5. Transfer rice and chicken to a serving platter and garnish with parsley. Enjoy.

Vegetarian Ratatouille

Original Recipe Yield 8 Servings

Ingredients:

- 3 garlic cloves, chopped
- 2 medium zucchini, chopped
- 1 medium onion, chopped
- 15 ounces canned tomatoes
- 1 cup all natural vegetable stock
- 1 medium green or red pepper, chopped
- 2 large eggplant, chopped into ½ inch squares
- 5 T olive oil
- Bay leaf
- Dried thyme
- Sea salt and pepper to taste

Directions:

1. Add oil and garlic to pan, cook until garlic is soft. Add onions and cook for 3 minutes. Add eggplant, zucchini, pepper, and stock. Cook until soft. Add tomatoes and season with salt and pepper.
2. Cook for 10 minutes on medium-low heat until flavors have blended.

Vegetarian Stuffed Bell Peppers

Original Recipe Yield 4 Servings

Ingredients:

- 4 medium bell peppers (.5 lb each)
- 1 ½ cups cooked rice (preferably organic)
- 3 T olive oil
- ½ cup onion, chopped
- 8 oz. marinara sauce
- 1 to 2 garlic cloves, chopped

Directions:

1. Cut the tops off the peppers and remove all the seeds. Chop up the pepper tops you've removed, chop into small pieces, and reserve. In a large pot of boiling water, parboil the peppers until just tender, 2 to 3 minutes. Remove with a slotted spoon and dry on paper towels.
2. In a large sauté pan or skillet, heat the oil over medium-high heat. Add the onions and chopped bell peppers and cook, stirring, until soft, about 3 minutes. Add the ground meat, garlic, oregano, salt, and pepper. Cook until the meat is browned, stirring with a heavy wooden spoon to break up the lumps, about 6 minutes. Add the rice and tomato sauce and stir well. Remove from the heat and adjust the seasoning, to taste.

3. Pour enough water into a baking dish to just cover the bottom, about 1/8 inch deep. Stuff the bell peppers with the rice mixture and place in the baking dish. Bake until the peppers are very tender and the filling is heated through, 25 to 30 minutes.
4. Remove from the oven and let rest for 10 minutes before serving.

Grilled Sirloin with Sautéed Broccoli Rabe

Original Recipe Yield 2 Servings

Ingredients:

- 2 12 oz. sirloin steaks (or
- 1 broccoli rabe bunch, chopped
- 3 T olive oil
- 2 garlic cloves, chopped
- Sea salt and pepper to taste
- 2 medium sweet potatoes

Directions:

1. Sirloin - Season sirloin steaks with salt and pepper and grill for approximately 7 minutes on each side or until desired cooking temperature.
2. Sweet Potatoes - Preheat oven to 400F. Microwave sweet potatoes on high for 5 minutes, on a plate. Wrap sweet potatoes in aluminum foil and transfer to oven. Cook at 400F for 15-20 minutes.
3. Broccoli Rabe - Add 3 T olive oil and chopped broccoli rabe unto large pan. Cook on medium heat for 5 minutes, stirring frequently. Add garlic, sea salt and pepper and cook for additional 3 minutes.
4. Serve and enjoy.

Simple Beef Stew

Original Recipe Yield 8 Servings

Ingredients:

- 1 ½ pounds lean cubed beef
- 4 T gluten free flour
- 1 dash paprika
- 1 gluten-free beef bouillon cube
- 2 teaspoons olive oil
- 4 carrots, 1 inch thick
- 2 potatoes, cubed
- 1 medium onion, chopped
- 1 medium green pepper chopped
- 15 oz. stewed tomatoes, canned with juices
- 15 oz. corn, canned with juices
- 1 t Worcestershire sauce
- ½ t salt
- ½ t pepper

Directions:

1. Dredge meat in flour, brown in hot oil.
2. Add meat and all other ingredients into Crock-Pot and cook on low for 6-8 hours or high for 2-4 hours.
3. Or cover and simmer on medium for 90 minutes.

Simple and Spicy Chili

Original Recipe Yield 6 Servings

Ingredients:

- 2 lbs. ground beef
- 1 large onion chopped
- 1 30 oz. can stewed tomatoes
- 2 packages gluten-free chili seasoning
- 1 medium green or red bell pepper, chopped
- 2 jalapeño peppers, diced

Directions:

1. Brown ground beef and drain grease.
2. Combine all ingredients in Crock-Pot, stir, and let cook 6 hours.
3. You can substitute ground turkey or buffalo/bison meat in this recipe too.

Spaghetti and Turkey Meatballs

Original Recipe Yield 6 Servings

Your favorite gluten-free sauce or

Sauce Ingredients:

- 1 large can crushed tomatoes
- 2 cloves of crushed garlic
- Minced onion
- 1 T olive oil
- Salt, pepper, oregano, and basil to taste.

Directions:

1. Sauté garlic and minced onion in olive oil.
2. Add crushed tomatoes and paste. Add crushed garlic. Let simmer while you make meatballs.

Meatballs Ingredients:

- 1 lb. ground turkey
- 2 te sea salt
- Pepper to taste
- 2 cloves crushed garlic
- ¾ cup gluten free breadcrumbs soaked in almond milk (or coconut or rice milk)
- 2 T olive oil

- 2 egg whites
- Italian spices

Directions:

1. Mix all ingredients together with hands.
2. Form small balls and drop into sauce, cover and simmer for approximately 1 hour, while stirring occasionally.
3. Serve over your favorite gluten-free pasta.

Greek Pasta with Tomatoes, Olives, and Spinach

Original Recipe Yield 6 Servings

Ingredients

- 2 (14.5 oz.) cans Italian-style diced tomatoes
- 10 oz. fresh spinach, washed and chopped
- 8 oz. of your favorite olives
- 2 garlic cloves, chopped
- 8 oz. penne brown rice pasta

Directions:

1. Cook the pasta in a large pot of boiling salted water until al dente.
2. Meanwhile, combine tomatoes, garlic, and olives in a large nonstick skillet. Bring to a boil over medium high heat. Reduce heat, and simmer 10 minutes.
3. Add spinach to the sauce; cook for 2 minutes or until spinach wilts, stirring constantly.
4. Add pasta and stir for 2 minutes. Serve and enjoy.

Dessert

Avocado Smoothie

Original Recipe Yield 4 Cups

Ingredients:

- 1 ripe avocado, halved and pitted
- 1 cup almond milk (you may also use rice or hemp)
- ½ cup vanilla yogurt
- 3 T honey
- 8 ice cubes

Directions:

1. Combine the avocado, milk, yogurt, honey, and ice cubes in a blender; blend until smooth.

This recipe is courtesy of loveinit on allrecipes.com

Turmeric and Pineapple – Nature's Natural Inflammatory

Original Recipe Yield 2 Servings

Ingredients:

- 2 cups fresh pineapple
- 1 t turmeric

Directions:

1. Slice or cube pineapple. Sprinkle turmeric over pineapple and mix together.
2. Chill in refrigerator for 20 minutes and serve.

Gluten-Free Fudge Brownies

Ingredients:

- 2/3 cup gluten-free baking mix (such as Bob's Red Mill All Purpose GF Baking Flour®)
- ½ cup cornstarch
- 1 cup white sugar
- 1 cup packed brown sugar
- ¾ cup unsweetened cocoa powder
- 1 t baking soda
- 2 eggs, beaten
- ¾ cup margarine, melted

Directions:

1. Preheat oven to 350 degrees F (175 degrees C), and grease an 8x8 inch square baking dish.
2. Stir together the gluten-free baking mix, cornstarch, white sugar, brown sugar, cocoa powder, and baking soda in a bowl, sifting with a fork to remove lumps. Pour in the eggs and melted margarine, and mix with a large spoon or electric mixer on low until the mixture forms a smooth batter, 3 to 5 minutes. Scrape the batter into the prepared baking dish.
3. Place a sheet of aluminum foil on the oven rack to prevent spills as the brownies rise then fall during baking. Bake until a toothpick inserted in the center of the brownies comes out clean, 40 to 45 minutes.

This recipe is courtesy of SCRIBEFORGOD on allrecipes.com

Flourless and Sugar-Free Almond Butter Cookies

Original Recipe Yield 16-24 Cookies

Ingredients:

- 1 cup almond butter
- 1 cup granular Stevia
- 1 T baking powder
- 1 T water
- 1 egg

Directions

1. Preheat oven to 350 degrees F.
2. Combine all ingredients and use a teaspoon to place on non-stick cookie sheet.

Bake for 8 minutes. Let cool and rest for 20 minutes.

Flourless and Sugar-Free Chocolate Cake

Original Recipe Yield One 8-inch Cake

Ingredients:

- 4 oz. fine-quality bittersweet chocolate
- 1 stick unsalted butter
- ¾ cup granulated Stevia
- 3 large eggs
- ½ cup unsweetened cocoa powder plus additional for sprinkling

Directions:

1. Preheat oven to 375 F. Butter an 8-inch round baking pan.
2. Chop chocolate into small pieces.
3. In a double boiler or glass bowl, set over a saucepan of slowly simmering water. Add chocolate and butter and stir together until fully melted and smooth.
4. Remove top of double boiler or bowl from heat and whisk sugar substitute into chocolate mixture.
5. Add eggs and whisk well. Sift ½ cup cocoa powder over chocolate mixture and whisk until just combined.
6. Pour batter into pan and bake in middle rack of oven for 25 minutes or until the top has formed a thin crust.
7. Remove cake and cool on a rack for 10 minutes. Turn upside down and onto a serving plate.
8. Dust cake with additional cocoa powder.